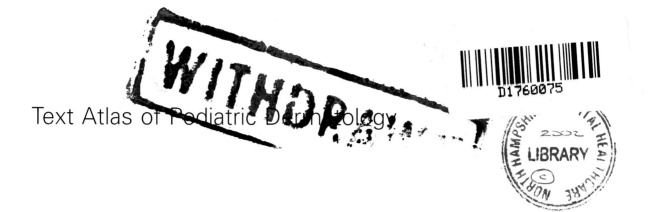

Text Atlas of Podiatric Dermatology

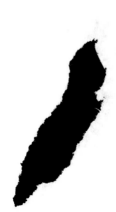

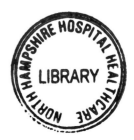

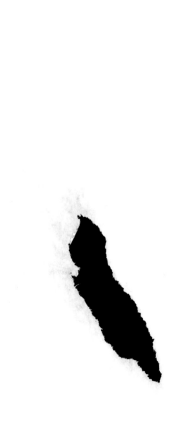

Text Atlas of Podiatric Dermatology

Rodney Dawber MA, MBChB, FRCP
Consultant Dermatologist
Churchill Hospital
Clinical Senior Lecturer in Dermatology
University of Oxford
Oxford, UK

Ivan Bristow BSc(Hons), MChS, PGCert
Senior Lecturer in Podiatry
University College Northampton
Northampton, UK

Warren Turner BSc(Hons), DPodM, MChS
Assistant Dean
School of Health & Community Studies
University of Derby
Derby, UK

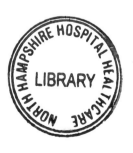
Martin Dunitz

© 2001 Martin Dunitz Ltd, a member of the Taylor & Francis group

First published in the United Kingdom in 2001
by Martin Dunitz Ltd, The Livery House, 7–9 Pratt Street, London NW1 0AE

Tel: +44 (0) 20 74822202
Fax: +44 (0) 20 72670159
E-mail: info@dunitz.co.uk
Website: http://www.dunitz.co.uk

Reprinted in paperback 2002

A CIP catalogue record for this book is available from the British Library

ISBN 1 84184 223 0

Distributed in the USA by
Fulfilment Center
Taylor & Francis
7625 Empire Drive
Florence, KY 41042, USA
Toll Free Tel.: +1 800 634 7064
E-mail: cserve@routledge_ny.com

Distributed in Canada by
Taylor & Francis
74 Rolark Drive
Scarborough, Ontario M1R 4G2, Canada
Toll Free Tel.: +1 877 226 2237
E-mail: tal_fran@istar.ca

Distributed in the rest of the world by
Thomson Publishing Services
Cheriton House
North Way
Andover, Hampshire SP10 5BE, UK
Tel: +44 (0) 1264 332424
E-mail: salesorder.tandf@thomsonpublishingservices.co.uk

Composition by 𝐓\ Tek-Art, Croydon, Surrey
Printed and bound in China by Imago

Contents

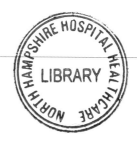

Preface

For many years there has been a very positive link between podiatry and clinical dermatology, but unfortunately they largely remain apart in most medical cultures, both in training and in practice. Where they have begun to overlap in the clinical treatment of foot dermatological problems the benefits rapidly become obvious to those involved. Good examples include the often better management of ingrowing toenail by the podiatrist and the advantages of dermatological training in the correct use of cryosurgery. The podiatrist has the great advantage of always knowing that foot problems are moving all the time (!) and are constantly modified and compounded by this; many dermatologists only see foot disease in static pathogenetic terms. Sometimes a skin or nail problem may be helped more by alleviating the effects of friction and pressure than by complex pharmacological agents. In reality both should be able to work together.

Because of the different training, aptitudes and attitudes of the various specialists dealing with toenail pathology, the authors have allowed some overlap in description of subjects such as nail anatomy and foot function — in an attempt to show where in one context static structural considerations are appropriate whilst in another a more functional attitude is required.

In producing this Text Atlas the authors sincerely hope that it will be useful to those dealing with foot skin problems whatever their current formal speciality training may be — as traditional medical speciality barriers 'break down' it would be wonderful to think, as we evidently do, that podiatrist, dermatologist, nurse and primary care physician could directly share their skills in a practical way.

Rodney Dawber
Ivan Bristow
Warren Turner

1 Anatomy and physiology of the skin

INTRODUCTION

During a lifetime the average foot travels many thousands of miles. With each footstep it absorbs the impact of around twice the body weight. Typically our feet go unnoticed for the majority of our lives, remaining covered and out of sight. When foot problems do arise, embarrassment often prevents the individual from seeking attention. From a medical point of view, the feet are rarely examined as routine practice. In clinical medical practice the foot is rarely examined routinely; rarely is it seen as a 'unit' with specific functional problems in health and disease. The skin overlying the foot is the body's main interface with the ground and so has subtle adaptations to its structure at other sites in order to fulfil this role. Dermatological disease of the foot is not uncommon and in the last few hundred years in advanced societies the use of footwear has added an extra dimension to skin pathology.

The functions of the skin are summarized in Table 1.1. (Those in italics are of particular importance to the foot). Figure 1.1 shows the major components of the skin.

Table 1.1   Summary of skin function

Barrier functions
   Physical: thermal/mechanical/radiation
   Chemical: irritants and allergens
   Biological: viral/fungal/arthropodal

Sensory functions
   Pain/temperature/touch/vibration

Other functions
   Thermoregulation
   Vitamin D production

ANATOMY

The skin is divided into two distinct layers, the *epidermis* and the *dermis*. Each layer has its own distinct structure, which when juxtaposed, provide the skin with the qualities needed to fulfil its function. Below these layers lie the subcutaneous tissue (hypodermis or sub-cutis), mainly composed of fat cells (lipocytes).

The *epidermis* (Figures 1.2a–c) of the foot, due to its contact with the ground, must maintain integrity to prevent infection or damage to deeper structures. It is the outermost layer of the skin and is composed of four or five different strata. Covering the whole surface of the foot, the epidermis is thickest on the weight bearing, glaborous plantar surface (around 1.5 mm; Figure 1.2b) and thinner on the dorsum (Figure 1.2c). The principle cells of the epidermis are the keratinocyte, Langerhan's cell and melanocyte.

The *basal layer* (*stratum germinativum*) consists of a regular, undulating layer of cuboidal keratinocytes. These undergo occasional division and the resulting cells move upwards into the higher layers of the epidermis.

In the *stratum spinosum* (syn: *prickle cell layer*), the cells adopt a more polyhedral shape and develop keratin filaments (tonofilaments) within their cytoplasm (Figures 1.2a–c). Some of the tonofilaments form spiny processes (desmosomes) which project outwards and meet with those of other adjacent cells. It is believed they form intercellular bridges which add resilience to the epidermis.

Individual cells are continually formed by mitotic cell division in the basal layer. These move up into the stratum spinosum and then into the *stratum granulosum*. At this level the cells have a more flattened appearance and inside the cell a number of changes occur. Keratohyalin granules appear within the cytoplasm and pack the cell, giving a granular

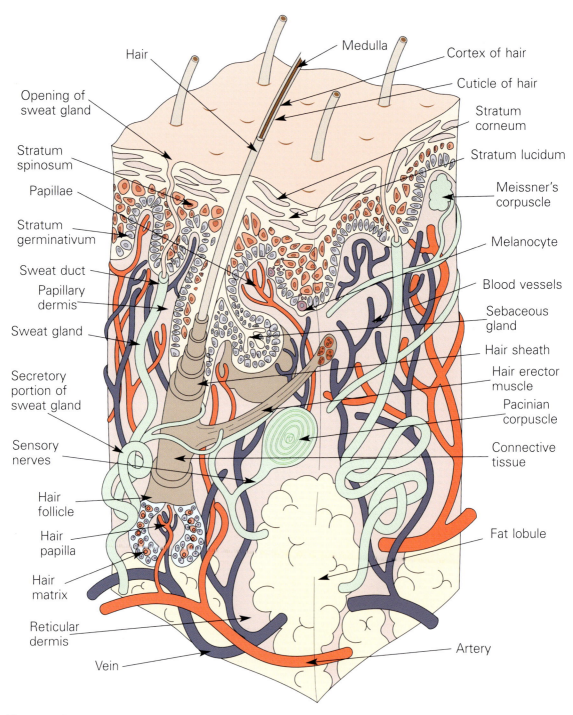

Figure 1.1
Anatomical features of the epidermis and dermis.

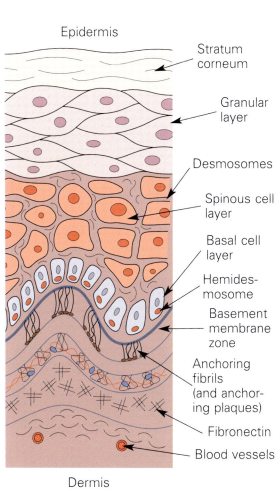

Epidermis

Stratum corneum

Granular layer

Desmosomes

Spinous cell layer

Basal cell layer

Hemides-mosome

Basement membrane zone

Anchoring fibrils (and anchoring plaques)

Fibronectin

Blood vessels

Dermis

(a)

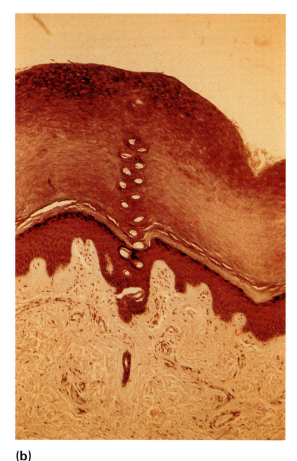

(b)

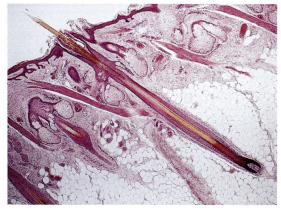

(c)

Figure 1.2
(a) Strata of the epidermis and dermis.
(b) Anatomy of the sole of the foot: thick stratum corneum with a sweat pore penetrating through it.
(c) Skin from dorsum of toe with relatively thin epidermis and a large hair follicle.

appearance, gradually 'engulfing' the tonofilaments. Lamellar granules are also synthesized by the cell at this level, and migrate to the cell membrane, expelling their contents into the inter-cellular spaces. It is thought these expelled lipid components are a major factor in skin permeability. This granular cell layer is the stage of 'cell death'; intracellularly degrading organelles can be seen.

At the level of the *stratum corneum* (horny layer), which is about 15–20 layers thick, the cells are flat, anucleate and packed with keratin. Gradually the upper cells of the stratum corneum detach and flake away, the process of desquamation.

On the plantar surface of the foot, an extra layer is visible microscopically in the epidermis, between the granular and horny layer — this is the stratum lucidium and it is only found on thick, glaborous (non-hairy) skin.

The epidermis can be considered a very active 'organ', constantly generating keratinocytes from its basal layer which, over a period of 28–46 days, ascend outwards and undergo a process of maturation, keratinization and desquamation. This process produces a regular turnover of cells throughout life and has an important physiological role.

Trauma, desiccation and maceration can break down the stratum corneum providing a portal of entry for infective organisms. However, with certain organisms, particularly fungi, it has been shown that the response to invasion leads to an increased activity, causing faster maturation and desquamation of the epidermal cells, effectively shedding the invading organism.

Throughout the basal layer are found specialist cells called melanocytes (Figure 1.3). These are dendritic cells which produce melanin in organelles called melanosomes. The melanin is evenly 'donated' as pigment granules to the surrounding keratinocytes, via the dendritic processes of the melanocytes. Melanin protects the skin against cell damage due to UV radiation. Exposure to such radiation causes the skin to darken and also stimulates further melanin production. The number of melanocytes in darker and lighter skinned individuals is similar; however, the melanin produced in dark skin is produced in much larger, more dense granules.

Changes in the level of pigmentation in skin can be induced by other factors. It has been postulated that the melanocyte has an important role in inflammation of the skin. Notably in darker skinned individuals, any form of inflammation in the skin can lead to hyperpigmentation or, less commonly, hypopigmentation. Pituitary hormones such as adrenocorticotrophic hormone and melanocyte stimulating hormone, other chemical mediators in the skin, can cause a similar effect. Melanocytes are distributed fairly evenly throughout the whole epidermis of the foot but as plantar skin is rarely exposed to UV radiation, it rarely shows any significant pigmentation.

The *Langerhan's cell* is another dendritic cell of the epidermis (Figure 1.3). They make up about 2–6 per cent of the cells in the epidermis and are found particularly around the stratum spinosum. They are derived from the bone marrow and are important in skin immunity, having antigen presenting functions similar to those of the macrophage. Furthermore, they promote T-cell proliferation. It is thought that they play an important role in lymphocyte-mediated allergic reactions.

The interface between the dermis and the epidermis is known as the dermo-epidermal junction. This is a basement membrane divided into three layers, crossed by fibrils and filaments and forming an anchoring surface between the dermis and epidermis (Figures 1.2a, 1.3). Pathologically, the dermo-epidermal junction is a cleavate plane for some blistering diseases.

Deep to the epidermis lies the dermis (Figure 1.1). This consists essentially of dense fibro-elastic tissues in a 'gel-like' base (ground substance) containing glycosaminoglycans. Tensile strength is provided by collagen

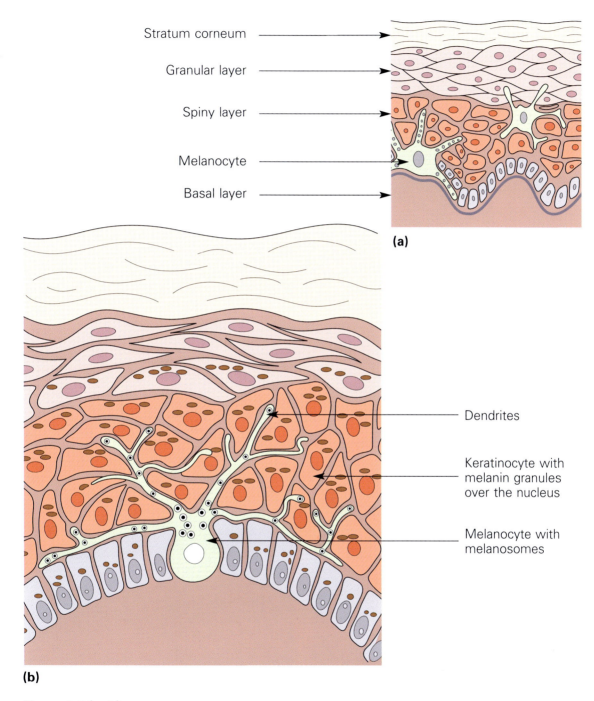

Figure 1.3 (a, b)

Melanin distribution and melanocytes in the epidermis: **(a)** Sites of melanocytes in basal and suprabasal areas; **(b)** migration of melanosomes along dendrites from where they are donated to adjacent keratinocytes (melanin granules).

strands, with elasticity afforded by interwoven elastic fibres.

At the dermo-epidermal junction, the dermis makes regular finger-like folds into the overlying epidermis called dermal papillae. These are complemented by 'protrusions' from the epidermis into the dermis known as rete or epidermal ridges/pegs. On the plantar surface, where there is increased mechanical stress, the dermal papillae and rete pegs reach much deeper hence a greater surface area is created between the two layers, forming a much stronger attachment.

The thin, upper layer of the dermis is known as the papillary dermis, while the deeper layer is the reticular dermis. The papillary layer contains most of the blood and lymphatic vessels, while the less vascular reticular layer possesses more dense collagen and elastic fibres. Cells of the immune system are present in the dermis, i.e. T-lymphocytes and mast cells.

The subcutaneous layer is a dense plane of primarily fat (adipose) and areolar tissue to which fibres from the dermis are firmly anchored. Over the sole of the foot the sub-

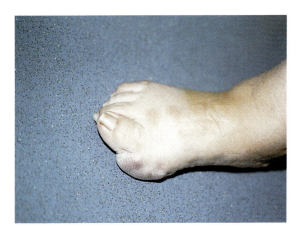

Figure 1.5
Medial displacement of FFP in patient with rheumatoid arthritis.

cutis is thickened, particularly over the weight bearing areas of the heel and metatarsal heads (up to 18 mm). Fatty tissue in the heel areas is divided by numerous fibrous septa which attach the dermis to the periosteum of the calcaneus. Across the plantar surface of the metatarsal heads it is more loosely attached to

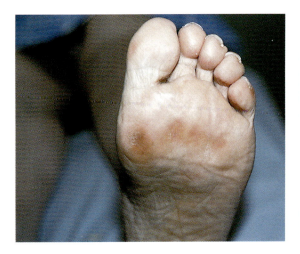

Figure 1.4
Early loss of fibro-fatty padding (FFP) across metatarsal heads.

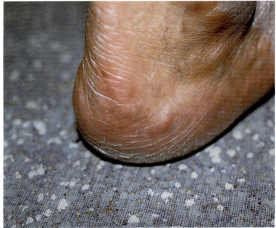

Figure 1.6
Solitary piezogenic papule arising on the heel.

surrounding tissue. Fat across the sole of the foot has an important protective role. Not only does it serve as a good insulator but the fibrous septae effectively form sealed chambers of fat. When subject to mechanical forces, fat flows within these chambers and act collectively as a fluid cushion absorbing the stresses of locomotion. Abnormalities of this fatty layer may give significant problems (Figures 1.4–1.6).

Clinically, herniations of this fatty tissue into the dermis may occur, particularly on the medial side of the heel (visible when standing). This condition is most prevalent in middle age patients. Occasionally, these herniations may give rise to pain around the heel area and as such, are termed painful piezogenic papules. Generalized atrophy of the fat pad can also arise with ageing and diabetes. In the forefoot, anterior migration of the fat pad may occur in rheumatoid disease.

BLOOD SUPPLY

The main blood supply to the skin (Figure 1.1) arises from a network of vessels located in the subcutaneous layer. At this lowest level branches supply eccrine sweat glands and hair follicles located deep in the reticular dermis. Vessels ascend from this network and fan out to form a second plexus in the mid-dermis. Arterioles from this level supply smaller hair follicles and their associated structures. Other vessels ascend further to form a third plexus in the papillary dermis. From the papillary plexus, single capillaries loop upwards into the dermal papillae. These tiny vessels loop and descend to drain into venules within the papillary plexus and then descend further into the deeper dermis, eventually reconnecting with the subcutaneous blood vessels.

The advantages of a layered system of blood vessels become obvious when considering the role of the skin in thermo-regulation. The sympathetic nervous system is able to direct blood flow by controlling vessel diameter; when blood is diverted to the most superficial layer, heat loss is at its greatest and when there is constriction of the superficial vessels blood flow is redirected through the deeper dermis so that much less heat is lost through convection and radiation via the epidermis. The foot, owing to its small surface area, has a limited role in thermo-regulation. The foot arterial supply to the skin is shown in Figure 1.7.

Within the papillary dermis are the lymphatic vessels which act as 'drains' for intercellular fluid and small particles within the dermis. At

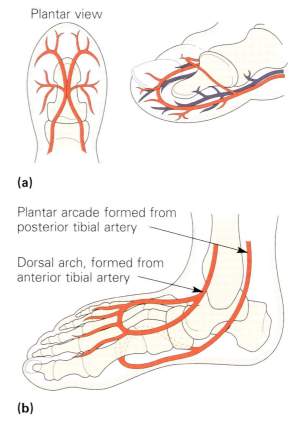

Plantar view

(a)

Plantar arcade formed from posterior tibial artery

Dorsal arch, formed from anterior tibial artery

(b)

Figure 1.7
Arterial supply of **(a)** the toe and **(b)** the foot.

the highest level in the dermis, lymphatic 'end bulbs' feed into larger lymphatic vessels which traverse deep into the dermis, connecting with the subcutaneous layer. The superficial vessels in their normal state are collapsed and highly permeable. Lymph drained from the lateral side of the foot flows up the leg into the popliteal lymph nodes behind the knee while the remainder of the lymph from the foot drains directly into the inguinal nodes of the thigh.

NERVE SUPPLY

Sensory perception is a vital component in maintaining skin integrity (see Chapter 3). The dermis is well supplied with nerves (both myelinated and unmyelinated fibres). In the foot, sensory nerves connect with the main pedal nerves. As with the rest of the body they are arranged in pattern of dermatomes (Figure 1.8).

The main sensations of the skin are tactile (touch, pressure and vibration), thermo-receptive (heat and cold) and nociception (pain and itch). Receptors in the skin vary in density according to their location, some being encapsulated, others being free (Figures 1.1, 1.9).

On the plantar surface where the papillary ridges are very dense and most organized (particularly on the heel, ball of the foot and volar surfaces of the toes) neural tissue is at its most orderly and dense. Numerous free nerve endings and Merkel's discs are present. These discs are of unknown origin but are located in the dermal papillae and are linked to local keratinocytes in the epidermis. Their function is thought to be that of tactile perception.

Meissner's corpuscles are oval structures containing neural and connective tissues. These occur in large numbers on the soles of the feet, particularly within the volar pads of the digits, protruding into the basal lamina at the dermo-epidermal junction. Their function is

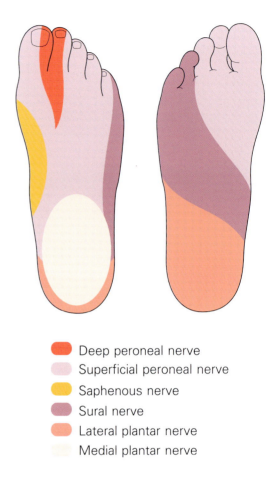

- ■ Deep peroneal nerve
- ■ Superficial peroneal nerve
- ■ Saphenous nerve
- ■ Sural nerve
- ■ Lateral plantar nerve
- □ Medial plantar nerve

Figure 1.8
Dorsal and plantar dermatomes.

thought to be that of touch perception. Deeper in the dermis are Pacinian corpuscles (pressure and vibratory receptors) close to the periosteum of the phalanges and extensively across the plantar surface.

Pain and itch perception (nociception) arises from the activation of free nerve endings at the dermo-epidermal junction and throughout the dermis. Nociceptors respond to multiple noxious sensations such as mechanical, chemical, hot and cold.

As the skin changes, from thick plantar skin to thinner hairy dorsal skin, the neural network

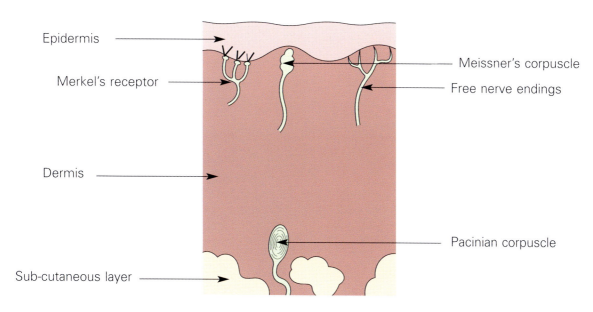

Figure 1.9
Relationship of the main sensory nerve endings found in the skin on the foot.

becomes less organized. Tactile receptors exist in the root hair plexuses, any movement of the hair shaft on the dorsum of the skin is detected by these receptors. Table 1.2 shows the main functions of the sensory nerve supply.

APPENDAGES

Hair follicles and their associated sebaceous and apocrine sweat glands are found on the dorsum of the foot (Figure 1.10). On the

Table 1.2 Summary of main nerve terminals found in the dermis of the foot.

Name	Location	Function
Meissner's corpuscle	Dermal papillae (particularly numerous in hands and feet)	Highly sensitive to light touch
Merkel's receptor	Dermal papillae	Sustained light touch
Pacinian corpuscle	Deep dermis/subcutaneous layer border (particularly in fat pads)	Vibratory perception
Free nerve endings	Dermal papillae and throughout dermis	Nociception (pain) thermoreception chemoreception

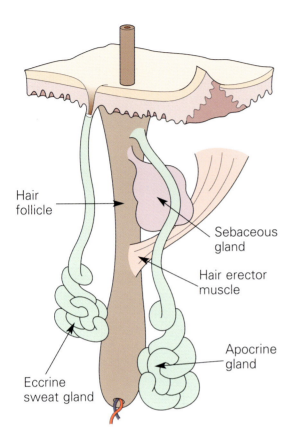

Figure 1.10
Hair follicle and associated structures.

plantar surface numerous eccrine (free) sweat glands are found (Figure 1.2b).

THE NAIL

The nail (Figure 1.11) has evolved as a tool to aid dexterity and the manipulation of small objects. However, in the foot the role of the toenail has lessened to that of offering protection of the underlying digital structure.

The hard keratinous nail plate arises from a group of specialist cells in the nail matrix, located at the base of the proximal nail fold,

(effectively an infolding of the epidermis). Here the nail plate is strongly attached to the nail bed and underlying phalanx by vertically orientated connective tissue fibres. The nail fold covers about a quarter of the plate, whilst the lateral edges meet with the epidermis to form the lateral nail folds or sulci.

The nail plate usually has a pale lunula (half-moon) visible at the proximal end. The lunula represents the most distal portion of the nail matrix, its colour being lighter than the more distal nail bed. Proximally, the eponychium (which arises as an outgrowth of the ventral surface of the proximal nail fold) and the cuticle act as effective seals to prevent infiltration by infection or irritants. More distally along the nail plate, prior to the nail separating from the nail bed at the hyponychium, is the onychodermal band (not always visible); this runs transversely across the nail bed. It is thought to be the most distal anchor for the nail plate.

The *nail plate* is a three layered structure composed of hard keratin, most of the plate being generated by the proximal and distal matrix. The deepest layer being added to the underside of the plate by the nail bed, distal to the lunula. Microscopically, the nail plate and nail bed fit together in a tongue-in-groove arrangement (Figure 1.11d).

Nail formation follows a similar sequence of events to that of the epidermis. Basal layer keratinocytes divide, differentiate and die, adding to the nail structure as it grows towards the end of the digit. Melanocytes are also found in small numbers in this matrix basal layer but normally their pigment is not visible in the nail plate.

The nail apparatus has a double blood supply (Figure 1.7). Lateral digital arteries run up the margins of the digits on the volar surface, close to the bone. Branches of these supply the phalanx and give rise to a superficial arcade which serves the proximal nail fold and matrix. Arteries then course dorsally, winding around the distal phalanx to just below the nail plate

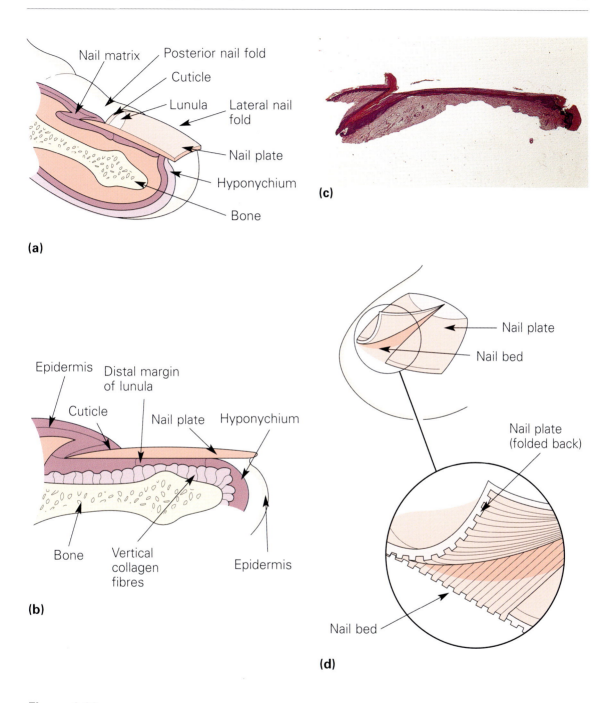

Figure 1.11

(a, b) Nail apparatus structures.

(c) Longitudinal nail biopsy, orientated to equate with **(b)**.

(d) Microscopic 'tongue in groove' nail bed and nail plate relationship.

giving rise to a proximal and distal arcade which serve the nail bed and matrix. Numerous muscular arterio-venous shunts (glomus bodies) exist in great numbers in the nail bed, their main role being to maintain an adequate blood supply to the nail apparatus in cold temperatures. Owing to its intricate neuro-vascular arrangement, changes in the general circulation and health are often reflected in the nail.

HAIR FOLLICLES AND ASSOCIATED STRUCTURES

Hair follicles are located over most of the body surface (Figures 1.1, 1.2c, 1.10). On the foot, they are restricted to the dorsum. Hair diseases which specifically affect the foot are rare.

Associated with the hair follicle is the sebaceous gland (Figure 1.10) which produces lipid rich sebum. Owing to their association with hairs, sebaceous glands are restricted to the dorsum of the foot and when compared to sebaceous glands in other areas of the body they are fairly inactive. Sebum production is stimulated by androgens, but inhibited by oestrogen.

Two types of sweat gland exist in the skin — eccrine and apocrine (Figures 1.1, 1.10). Eccrine glands are coiled structures located in the reticular dermis with a single duct ascending to an opening to the epidermis. They are most numerous on the sole of the foot. Apocrine glands are the larger of the two glands and are exclusively associated with hair follicles mainly in the inguinal and axilla areas and the areola of the breasts; they appear to have little significance on the foot. Sweat is a mixture of water, sodium chloride, urea, ammonia and other chemicals. Its release is controlled by sympathetic branches of the autonomic nervous system. Over the whole body, sweating acts as a cooling mechanism by its evaporation and could also be seen as an excretory function. Sweat glands in the foot, however, play little part in thermo-regulation; they produce a steady flow of sweat across the plantar surface, which serves to enhance grip. Sweat also helps to moisten the skin and when mixed with skin squames and the natural epidermal flora, a cocktail is formed which presents an inhospitable environment for most pathogenic organisms!

Across the sole of the foot, congenital flexure lines or skin creases are evident as a result of the arrangement of the collagenous fibres within the dermis. This pattern of dermatoglyphics is unique to each individual and remain unchanged throughout life. Dermatoglyphics are most prominent as a network of ridges over the main weight bearing surfaces — the heel, across the ball and the plantar aspects of the toes. Interestingly, as dermatoglyphics become exaggerated over the weight bearing areas of the plantar surface, clinically one is able to gauge where most of the weight is being borne by examination. It is thought that their function in the foot is twofold. Firstly, they enhance tactile sense across the skin. This theory is backed up by the fact that cutaneous sensory nerve endings are more densely congregated in areas of prominent dermatoglyphics. Secondly, the pattern of ridges is somewhat analogous to that of the tread of a tyre. This in conjunction with moderate amounts of sweat, serves to enhance the grip of the toes and sole by increasing the friction co-efficient.

2 Assessment of skin and foot function

INTRODUCTION

In many ways foot abnormalities require assessment with exactly the same principles as those at other sites. However, the movements of the foot in the gait cycle and the effects of footwear almost always alter podiatric dermatological disorders.

SKIN ASSESSMENT

As with any skin disease, careful assessment is the key to making an accurate diagnosis. One is then able to plan and instigate the most appropriate form of treatment for the presenting condition. The assessment process can be considered in four stages:

(i)   history taking
(ii) physical examination
(iii) assessment of foot function
(iv) special/further investigations.

Three of these can be seen as those used for dermatological assessment in general. The functional assessment illustrates the various dynamic mechanisms since these play a role in skin diseases of the foot. Often the skin is assessed in a 'static' manner but dynamics and foot shape are important factors in the disease process. Many diseases of the foot skin are caused directly by functional faults. Other disorders may be altered by variations in foot shape or movement: this includes diseases of the skin in general that are altered by the nature of foot skin, its movements in the gait cycle, and factors such as footwear, friction and pressure effects.

History taking

Taking a detailed history is a very important process. Accurate and clearly written notes regarding the distribution and extent of lesions provides a good baseline for any further comparison at a later stage. In this way a systematic approach is a good technique to adopt; this focuses one's practice and provides a clear record of the condition and simplifies interspecialty communication.

There is no single fixed questioning technique in history taking since there are many skin disorders that affect the foot; however, in general, specific areas of questioning may act as a good basic guide. These include:

- The patient's age and sex.
- The patient's own history, including the duration and course of the disease.
- Itching (pruritus) or pain arising from the eruption should be recorded together with any known precipitating factors. Common causes of localized itching on the foot include lichen planus, tinea pedis and dermatitis/eczema.
- Previous medical history. Are there any underlying systemic factors which may predispose to this condition? Is there a history of skin disease?
- Current or previous medication (local or systemic). Note in particular any previous treatments for the presenting complaint and their effects.
- Family history, particularly of any skin disease.
- Social history. Note should be taken of the patients occupation/leisure activities, sports, etc.; particularly note if there has been any recent change in the patient's normal or regular activities.
- Footwear. It is good practice for the patient to bring their most frequently worn shoes for assessment. Has there been any change in the type of footwear worn recently?

PHYSICAL EXAMINATION

When examining the foot, it is pertinent to assess footwear. Not all skin diseases are caused by it, but many are exacerbated by footwear whether of good or of poor quality.

Examination of the feet is best conducted initially with the leg exposed to the knee. If there is reasonable suspicion of other lesions then other areas of the body should be examined. Dermatological disease may produce a wide variety of lesions on the skin and due to this diversity, dermatology has derived its own specific terminology to describe skin lesions:

- **Site(s) and/or distribution**
  This can be very helpful: for example, psoriasis has a predilection for the knees, elbows, scalp and lower back; eczema favours the flexures in children.

Table 2.1 Assessment of the foot.

Glossary of terms

Flat lesions
Erythema: an area of redness over the skin.
Macule: a flat area of local discolouration within the skin.
Patch: a term to describe a macule greater than 1 cm in diameter.

Raised/palpable lesions
Papule: a raised area, nodular in form less than 5 mm across.
Plaque or disc: a flat raised lesion.
Nodule: a papule larger than 5 mm in diameter.

Lesions due to fluid accumulation
Vesicle: a small blister (less than 5 mm across).
Bulla: a blister larger than 5 mm across.
Pustule: a pus filled vesicle or bulla.
Wheal: a raised transitory, compressible area of dermal oedema (colour usually red or white).

Vascular lesions
Haematoma: a collection of blood under the skin or nail.
Purpura: a discolouration of the skin due to extravasation of blood into the skin.
Telangiectasia: a visible, dilated capillary.

Other lesions
Scale: an accumulation of stratum corneum, which easily detaches.
Fissure: a small split in the skin which may/may not extend into the epidermis.
Crust: dried exudate present on the skin surface.
Hyperkeratosis: a thickening of the stratum corneum.
Horn: an elevated projection of keratin.
Lichenification: a flat-topped thickening of the skin often secondary to scratching.
Maceration: an appearance of surface softening due to constant wetting.
Excoriation: a secondary, superficial ulceration, due to scratching.
Atrophy: reduction or thinning of the epidermis and/or dermis.
Ulcer: a total loss of an area of epidermis extending into the dermis.

- **Characteristics of individual lesions**

  The type. Table 2.1 lists the most common and important terms and their definitions.

  The size, shape, outline and border. Size is best measured, rather than being compared to various known objects. Lesions may be various shapes, e.g. round, oval, annular. Linear or 'irregular'; straight edges and angles may suggest external factors. The border is well defined in psoriasis, but blurred in most patches of eczema.

  The colour. It is always useful to note the colour, i.e. red, purple, brown, slate-black, etc.

  Surface features. It is helpful to assess whether the surface is smooth or rough, and to distinguish crust (dried serum) from scale (hyperkeratosis); some assessment of scale can be helpful, e.g. 'silvery' in psoriasis.

  The texture — superficial? deep? Use your fingertips on the surface; assess the depth and position in or below the skin; lift scale or crust to see what lies beneath; try to make the lesion blanch with pressure.

- **Secondary sites**

  Look for additional features which may assist in diagnosis, such as:
  - the nails in psoriasis
  - the fingers and wrists in scabies
  - the toe-webs in fungal infections
  - the mouth in lichen planus.

- **Special techniques**

  These will be covered in the appropriate chapters, but include:
  - scraping a psoriatic plaque for capillary bleeding
  - the Nicolsky sign in blistering diseases, i.e. on pressing an intact blister, the latter extends at the margins (as in pemphigus)
  - 'diascopy' in suspected cutaneous tuberculosis, i.e. 'apple jelly' granulomas seen through glass pressed on the lesion.

A basic sketch in the notes is a good way to highlight the distribution of lesions and their relative size. When describing lesions, their

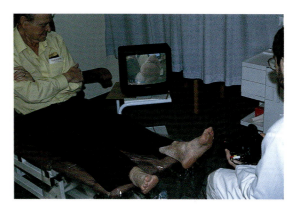

Figure 2.1

Video equipment enables objective recording of static and functional signs in foot problems to be made.

arrangement/pattern should be noted, i.e. linear, annular (ring like), clustered or symmetrical. In general, lesions with a symmetrical pattern arise as a result of a systemic (or internal) condition: while a unilateral spread or marked asymmetry may indicate external influences such as infection. Irritant or allergic contact dermatitis may arise symmetrically, correlating to areas where the irritant or allergen is in contact with the skin. Certain disorders show the Koebner phenomenon — in diseases such as psoriasis and lichen planus, the disorder may appear on previously healthy skin when subjected to trauma, i.e. physical damage such as scratching or friction.

If the eruption occurs in other areas of the body, note should be made of the specific sites affected, e.g. scalp, flexures or extensor surfaces.

The use of photography or video equipment may add objective, recorded evidence and allow the patients with poor mobility/eyesight to visualise and appreciate the foot problem (Figure 2.1). Follow up recordings may be taken for further comparison.

Sweat gland function

Assessment of the skin may reveal evidence of sweat gland faults (Table 2.2) i.e.:

- very dry skin; anhidrosis (Figure 2.2)
- excessive production of sweat, *hyperhidrosis* (Figure 2.3).

Table 2.2 Causes of anhidrosis and hyperhidrosis of the foot.

Anhidrosis (lack of sweating)

Damage to neurological pathways
Diabetes mellitus
CNS disorders
Leprosy

Displacement of sweat ducts
Psoriasis
Eczema
Lichen planus
Miliaria

Lack or loss of sweat glands
Damage/scarring to areas of the skin
Congenital lack of sweat glands
(ectodermal dysplasia)

Hyperhidrosis (excessive sweating)
Physiological – normal in young adults
Emotions
Stress
Endocrine disorders (i.e. hypoglycaemia,
hyperthyroidism)
CNS disorders
May be associated with certain palmo-plantar
keratodermas and Raynaud's phenomenon

In severe cases of anhidrosis cracking and fissuring of the epidermis may occur, particularly around the heel, with painful calloused borders. Deep fissuring may extend into the dermis and be associated with recurrent bleeding.

Hyperhidrosis, when symmetrical, is most commonly associated with young active individ-

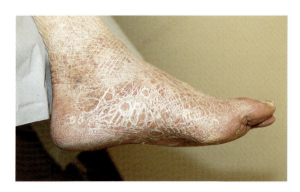

Figure 2.2
Anhidrosis of the foot.

uals after puberty; it is usually physiological rather than pathological (Figure 2.4). Resolution generally occurs by the third decade – sweat production normally decreases with age. In hyperhidrosis, sweat secretion may increase to such an extent that the skin becomes very hydrated and macerated, particularly if the footwear/hosiery is occlusive. Moist fissuring may develop between the toes and blistering may occur on the plantar surface. At this stage secondary bacterial or fungal infection can occur generating unpleasant odour and even brown discolouration to the skin (bromhidrosis).

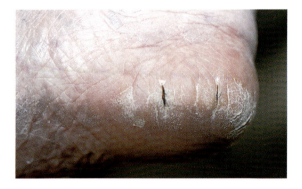

Figure 2.3
Anhidrosis of the foot with heel fissuring. Dry skin associated with the forces of weight-bearing may lead to tissue breakdown.

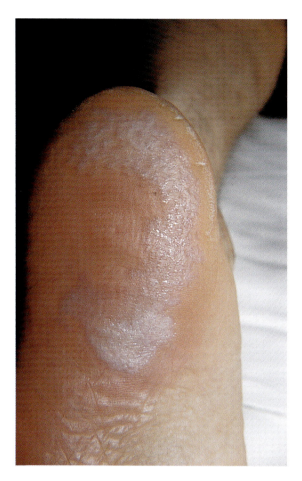

Figure 2.4
Hyperhidrosis of the sole of the foot.

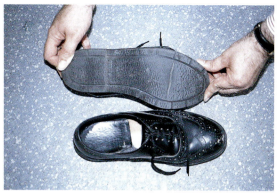

Figure 2.5
Assessment of footwear is an important part of examination. Footwear that is badly worn or ill-fitting may exacerbate skin problems.

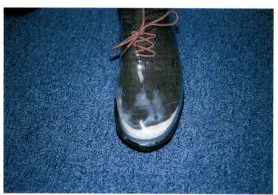

Figure 2.6
A plastic shoe highlights how occlusion can increase humidity within the shoe.

Footwear assessment

Footwear is often overlooked as a contributory factor in skin and nail disease of the foot (Figures 2.5, 2.6). The main causes of footwear related conditions arise as a result of:

• poor fitting
• inadequate design or construction
• excessive wear to shoes.

Where peripheral neuropathy or ischaemia exist the effect of these problems is often amplified considerably (see Chapter 3).

Poor fitting can be a result of too high heels, lack of a suitable fastening or inadequate shape in relation to the patient's foot. These problems may cause undue pressure to the epidermis or nail structures leading to considerable friction and shearing stresses on these areas. Most common pressure lesions are observed around the forefoot because shoes are often too narrow in this area. Shoes which are too large can cause compensatory clawing of the toes and gait alterations which can have similar effects.

The wearing of footwear constructed using occlusive materials such as plastic, rubber or synthetic fabric in 'the uppers' can lead to increase sweat accumulation and a rise in local humidity. This promotes the growth of pathogenic organisms, particularly fungi. Another factor with regard to footwear and its relation to foot problems is the amount of time a patient is active (standing, walking, running, etc.); this can affect the severity of virtually any pathology.

When feeling the inside surface of shoes, one can often find pressure areas as palpable dents or tears in the lining of the upper. A small mirror placed in the shoe is a good method of checking the uppers for signs of rubbing or excessive wear; it also illustrates to the patient the effect that footwear is having on the feet.

As part of the basic foot assessment, checking the arterial and venous circulation (Figures 2.7, 2.8) is a straightforward and informative test. The two main arteries serving the foot are the dorsalis pedis and the posterior tibial (Figures 2.7, 2.8). Whilst palpating the pulses the temperature of the skin may be noted, paying particular attention to the gradient up the foot and the leg and comparing the two limbs. Any local increases in temperature may indicate areas of inflammation. When pulses are not palpable due to swelling, or if poor arterial supply is suspected, an ankle/brachial pressure index may be taken by Doppler ultrasound and ankle cuff to give an objective analysis (Figure 2.9). This technique measures the systolic brachial and ankle blood pressure and is calculated by dividing the ankle pressure by the brachial pressure. A normal result would be 1.0. Readings less than this may indicate peripheral ischaemia; further vascular investigations should therefore be undertaken.

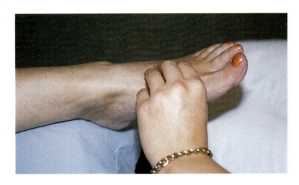

Figure 2.7
Palpating the dorsalis pedis artery.

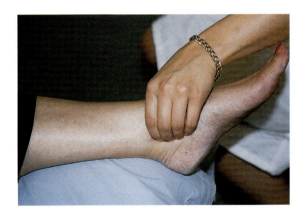

Figure 2.8
Palpating the posterior tibial artery.

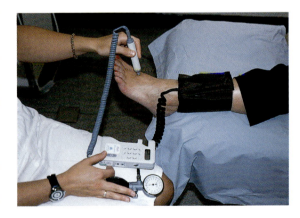

Figure 2.9
Assessing the ankle-brachial arterial index.

Sensory assessment may reveal areas of skin which are insensitive, a problem which is most common in patients with co-existing systemic diseases such as diabetes mellitus. Testing of sensation may include:

- light touch/protective sensation using monofilaments (Figure 2.10) or cotton wool
- hot/cold perception
- vibratory perception — this can be assessed with a tuning fork or by neurothesiometry.

Deficits in these areas should be noted and in some cases it may be possible to accurately map out areas of insensitivity. If areas of sensory deficit are found, detailed neurological testing is mandatory.

Table 2.3 Principal causes of toe nail disorders.

Traumatic (acute or chronic) — physical
                                       — chemical
Infection (local/systemic)
Dermatological disease
Systemic disease
Tumours
Congenital/genetic
Drug side effects/reactions

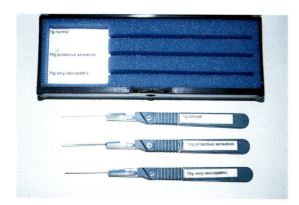

Figure 2.10
A set of sensory monofilaments.

Nail examination

Nail changes may occur as a result of many factors, these are summarized in Table 2.3. Fingernails should also be examined. Attention should be paid to the:

- Pattern of the affected nails
  - one foot/both feet
  - symmetry of pattern
  - number of nails affected
  - any fingernail involvement?
- Colour of the nail plate/nail bed/lunula.
- Thickness and texture of the nail plate.
- Nail shape – any abnormal longitudinal or transverse curvature.
- Attachment of the plate to the nail bed — noting any loosening distally or proximally.
- Surrounding structures. Noting any surrounding swelling, colour change, discharge etc.
- The presence of any pain in the toenail area should be noted describing whether it is constant or intermittent; or related to particular activity or footwear.

FOOT FUNCTION

For normal gait it is necessary for the foot to exhibit the following characteristics:

- adaption to changing terrain
- shock absorption
- provision of a stable base for propulsion.

The above characteristics might appear conflicting and contradictory but in fact, the foot displays certain of these characteristics at specific points of the gait cycle. The gait cycle is explained in Figure 2.11.

At heel strike, it is necessary for the foot to begin to absorb the shock of ground impact. If impact shock is not absorbed, the reaction forces are transmitted up the limb and may cause knee, hip or back problems. The foot

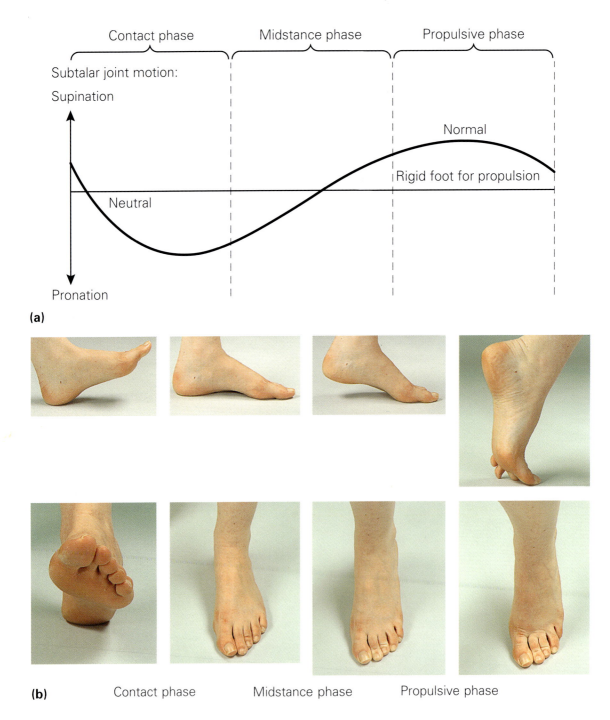

Figure 2.11
(a, b) The positions of the foot during normal gait cycle.

therefore acts as a shock absorber by deforming in relation to ground reaction forces. The central component of this deformation is the sub-talar joint. Upon heel strike, the sub-talar joint pronates causing eversion, dorsiflexion and abduction of the foot. This motion is decelerated by the tibialis anterior and posterior muscles, ensuring effective shock absorption.

Pronation of the sub-talar joint also 'unlocks' the mid-tarsal joints, creating a flexible forefoot. This is important when the forefoot comes into ground contact to ensure that the foot adapts to alterations in walking surface. This flexibility of the foot normally remains until the heel begins to leave the ground, just prior to propulsion. Abnormally pronated feet appear as flat feet with low medial longitudinal arches, medial bulging and eversion of the heel with bowing of the Achilles tendon (pes planus; Figure 2.12).

The propulsive phase of gait requires the foot to assume the properties of a rigid level. Loss of mid-tarsal flexibility is therefore required. The tibialis anterior and posterior muscles therefore contract, supinating (adducting, plantar flexing and inverting) the sub-talar joint. Body weight is transferred to the first ray and propulsion normally takes place through the hallux. The supinated foot acts as a stable base for this propulsive effect. Abnormally supinated feet appear as high arched feet with high medial longitudinal arches, retracted toes and high plantar pressure beneath the first and fifth metatarsal heads and the heel (pes cavus; Figure 2.12).

Failure of the foot to act either as an effective shock absorber or a rigid lever often results in secondary pathology. Trauma result-

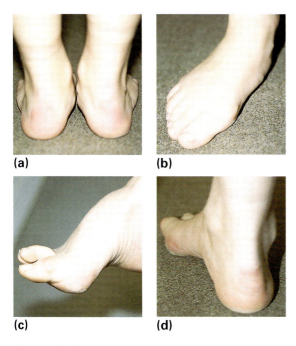

(a)

(b)

(c)

(d)

Figure 2.12

Features that may accompany a pronated and a supinated foot.
(a, b) Pronated (flat foot/pes planus): calcaneum everted, low arch, flexible or rigid foot, adductovarus toes, medial bulging of talar head, callus under second, third and fourth metatarsal heads.
(c, d) Supinated (high arched foot/pes cavus): calcaneum inverted, high arch, rigid foot, clawed or retracted toes, prominent extensor tendons, callus under 1st and 5th metatarsal heads.

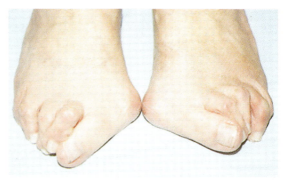

Figure 2.13

Hallux abductovalgus: rotation of the digit places extra pressure around the nail.

ing from abnormal pronation or supination usually affects the skin, particularly causing hyperkeratotic skin lesions. Trauma to the nail apparatus resulting from abnormal foot motion can result in nail hypertrophy, deformation or lysis. Long-term functional foot abnormalities can result in joint deformity of the foot. Typical deformities arising secondary to abnormal foot function include hallux abducto-valgus (Figure 2.13), hammer toe (Figure 2.14), hallux rigidus (Figure 2.15) and ankle equinus. These deformities can result in abnormal pressure, shear and friction acting on the skin which can in turn result in corns, calluses, blisters, ulcers. Table

2.4 summarizes skin and nail disorders which can be caused by abnormal foot function.

Table 2.4 Skin and nail disorders caused by abnormal foot function.

Skin disorders	Nail disorders
Friction blisters/ haemorrhage	Onychauxis
Bursitis	Sub-ungual haematoma
Corns	Involution
Callosities	Onycocryptosis
Fissures	Paronychia
Furrows	Distally embedded toenail
Bruises	Longitudinal splitting
Ulcers	Onycholysis

Assessment of the skin of the foot should therefore include reference to foot function in virtually all skin and nail disorders. Simple functional assessment of the foot should include the following:

- static non-weight-bearing evaluation
- static weight-bearing evaluation
- dynamic gait analysis.

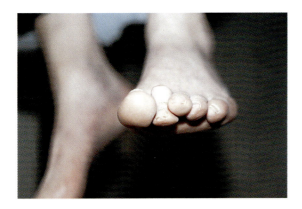

Figure 2.14
Hammer toe.

Static non-weight-bearing evaluation

Assessment of the foot and lower limb should be undertaken with the patient lying on a flat couch. The key aspects of the non-weight-bearing evaluation are:

1. Assessment of joints (hip, knee, ankle, subtalar, mid-tarsal, metatarsophalangeal, toes)
   — range of motion (normal, excessive, reduced)
   — direction of motion (normal, abnormal)
   — quality of motion (normal, crepitus, painful, restricted, etc.)
   — symmetry of motion (differences between right and left feet).

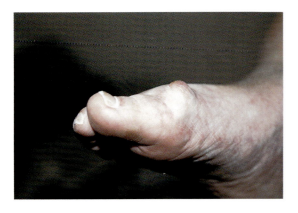

Figure 2.15
Hallux rigidus (syn.: limitus).

2. Positional abnormalities
   — fixed joint deformity (e.g. hammer toe, hallux valgus)
   — rear foot-sub-talar position (supinated, pronated, neutral)
   — forefoot to rear foot relationship (inverted, everted, neutral).
3. Foot morphology (Figure 12)
   — cavoid foot (high arch, retraction of toes)
   — pes planus foot (low arch, calcaneal eversion)
   — rectus foot (long, thin foot)
   — splay foot (short, wide foot – especially forefoot)
   — foot length non-weight-bearing
   — foot width non-weight-bearing.

Static weight-bearing examination

The foot should be examined with the patient standing in his/her normal 'relaxed' angle and base of gait (Figures 2.16–2.18). To achieve this stance position, ask the patient to walk on the spot. Without prior warning ask the patient to stop walking. The position the feet adopt at this stop position should represent the patient's

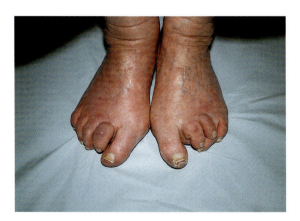

Figure 2.16

Toe deformity due to osteoarthritis.

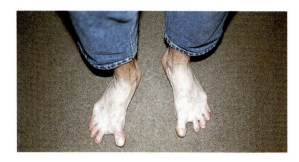

Figure 2.17

Hallux varus: the result of 'failed' hallux valgus surgery.

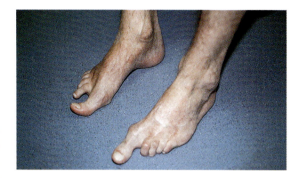

Figure 2.18

Retracted lesser toes have led to an excessively long, 'exposed' first toe.

normal angle and base of gait. Several indicators of foot function can be assessed from the patient's angle and base of gait position.

Calcaneal position

With the patient in this relaxed position, is the posterior aspect of the calcaneus inverted or everted? Eversion indicates a pronated sub-talar joint, inversion represents a supinated sub-talar joint. Severe pronation can cause bowing of the Achilles tendon (Helbing's sign).

Arch height

Are the patient's medial longitudinal foot arches too high, too low or normal? A very low arch height is associated with a pes planus foot type and excess sub-talar joint pronation (Figure 2.12). A very high arch height is associated with sub-talar joint supination and a cavoid foot type.

Digital position

The toes of the foot in static stance should bear weight along their entire plantar surface. Retraction or hammering of the toes will alter plantar weight-bearing. This often results in the toes bearing additional weight at the apices of the toes, and may result in retrograde trauma to the nail apparatus.

Foot size

A foot measure should be used to assess the length and width of the foot whilst weight-bearing. An excessively flexible or pronated foot can gain the equivalent of two shoe sizes in length from a non-weight-bearing to a weight-bearing position. Similarly, lax ligaments or excessive pronation/flexibility of the foot can cause increases in foot width when weight-bearing.

Dynamic weight-bearing assessment

Assessment of the patient's gait is invaluable in determining normal or abnormal foot function. Gait analysis also allows mechanical stresses on the skin and joints to be more easily identified. Assessment of the patient's gait often includes observation of walking and/or running, and assessment of plantar pressure distribution:

Assessment of walking

The most simple form of gait analysis involves observation of the patient walking unshod up and down a room or long corridor (Figure 2.11). It is important that the patient's gait is not impeded by rolled up trouser legs, etc., therefore he/she should ideally be wearing shorts. The patient should be encouraged to walk at his/her own pace, and given time to acclimatise to these instructions and observation. The clinician should observe the following:

- position of head and shoulders — symmetry, shoulder drop
- back position — excessive curvature, asymmetry
- pelvis function — effect of gluteal muscles, Trendelenberg sign
- hip motion — symmetry, range of motion
- knee function — range of motion, patella position, symmetry
- ankle position — range of motion, symmetry
- sub-talar joint motion — position of posterior calcaneal bisection at heel strike, forefoot loading, toe-off, signs of excessive pronation or supination
- mid-tarsal joint function — shape of lateral border of foot, medial bulging
- metatarsophalangeal and interphalangeal joints — toe motion, range of motion
- muscle and tendon phasic activity — overuse of tendons, stress of tendons/muscle
- pain — note any details of pain reported by the patient.

More complex forms of gait analysis may involve the use of video cameras and treadmills. High speed video recordings enable the patient's gait to be viewed in extreme slow motion, permitting more accurate determination of joint position and foot function.

Measurement of plantar pressure distribution

The distribution of mechanical forces on the plantar surface of the foot can have significant consequences for the quality of the skin and appendages. Excessive concentrations of pressure, shear and friction can result in the skin and nail pathologies described in Table 2.4. Techniques have been developed to assess the relative distribution of pressure on the plantar surface of the foot. These tests are useful to identify areas of the foot at risk of pressure induced lesions, including corns, calluses, blisters and ulcers. Plantar pressure measurement is also useful to predict the effect of mechanical therapy (e.g. insoles, padding etc.) on existing lesions. Simple techniques for plantar pressure measurement include rubber ink mats. The mats are inked and paper placed over the mat. The patient is instructed to walk over the mat. The pressure exerted by the patient weight-bearing on the mat is transferred to the paper to produce an ink footprint. Some mats (e.g. Harris and Beath mat) have deforming rubber ridges which produce more intense localised ink imprints over higher pressure areas.

More sophisticated plantar pressure systems make use of pressure transducer force plates linked to a computer. These systems are useful in quantifying the amount of vertical pressure present at specific parts of the foot. High pressure areas identified by the system are highly predictive of high risk areas for skin lesions.

FURTHER READING

Tollafield D, Merriman L (1995) *Assessment of the locomotor system.* In: *Assessment of the Lower Limb*, eds Merriman L, Tollafield D, (Edinburgh, Churchill Livingstone).

West S (1995) *Methods of analysing gait.* In: *Assessment of the Lower Limb*, eds Merriman L, Tollafield D (Edinburgh, Churchill Livingstone).

3 Skin disorders

INTRODUCTION

Many general skin diseases and systemic disorders have very specific symptoms and signs in their involvement of the foot. It is very important to recognize the signs affecting the feet since they may at times be limited to the feet; also, in recognizing these signs one should remember their general and systemic possibilities in podiatric practice when taking a history and examining the skin signs away from the feet. The treatment of diseases affecting the feet may be very different if there is widespread skin involvement.

HYPERKERATOTIC DISORDERS

Hyperkeratosis is the term used to describe the sign in which thickening of the outermost layer of the epidermis, the stratum corneum, is the main change. Causes can be due to a number of reasons including congenital and hereditary disorders, mechanical forces, skin disease, and various infections. Hyperkeratosis is probably the most common disorder affecting the foot. It may present as a primary lesion such as a callosity or as a secondary lesion to other diseases, i.e. eczema or psoriasis. This section will focus primarily on the disorders which give rise to hyperkeratosis as the primary lesion.

The thickness of the stratum corneum is governed by the rate of basal cell division in generating new epidermal cells; and the speed at which cells differentiate in the stratum spinosum, die and desquamate from the surface of the epidermis. Hyperkeratosis itself is the skin's natural response to intermittent friction or pressure; however, it may be considered pathological if it becomes symptomatic (due to excessive build up) or if it arises due to factors other than mechanical stress.

Mechanical causes: callosity and corns

The skin is well adapted to resist the external forces of friction and shear. However, when skin is subjected to chronic friction, initially an area of erythema develops and subsequently an increase in activity and hyperkeratosis occurs. Histologically, other changes occur such as increased local fibroblast activity, elongation of the rete pegs and thickening of the stratum spinosum. Areas of hyperkeratosis appear as rather 'rigid' yellow-coloured areas. The type of physical force that the skin is subjected to determines the type of primary lesion, i.e. corn or callosity (Figures 3.1–3.4). These are the commonest lesions seen affecting the foot, increasing in frequency with age. Depending on their cause, lesions may be single or multiple, symmetrical or asymmetrical. Table 3.1 summarizes the common causes of callosity and corns:

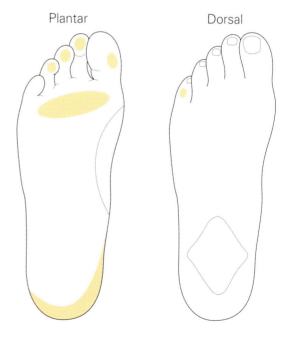

Figure 3.1

Common sites for callosity formation.

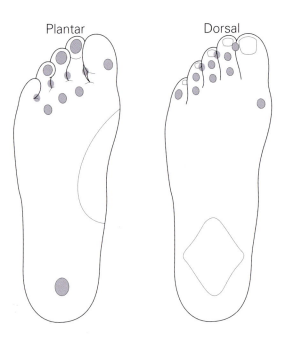

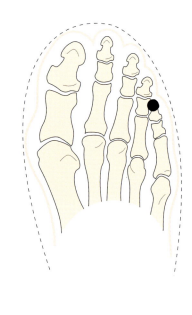

Figure 3.2

Common sites for hard corn formation.

Figure 3.3

Mechanism for inter-digital corn formation.

Table 3.1 Common causes of callosity and corns.

Footwear	Excessive wear
	Poor design
	Poor fit
Walking surface	Hyperkeratosis is common in those who spend prolonged periods of time standing, particularly on hard surfaces
Digital deformity/bone malalignment	Hallux valgus/rigidus
	Hammer/claw/retracted toes
Displacement or lack of fibro-fatty padding	Causes include ageing, long term steroid therapy, rheumatic diseases
Altered foot and leg biomechanics	This may result in higher pressures on specific areas of the foot
Weight gain/pregnancy	
Peripheral oedema	This may increase pressure from footwear as the feet swell

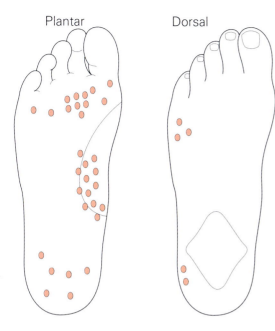

Plantar Dorsal

Figure 3.4
Common sites for seed corn formation.

Callosity (callous, callus, tylosis)

This is a diffuse area of hyperkeratosis (often of even thickness) caused by mechanical forces, most prevalent on areas of the foot exposed to intermittent pressure or friction (Figures 3.5–3.9). Though often asymptomatic, these lesions may give rise to a local burning or painful sensation when walking or standing. Callus is most commonly found on the plantar surface and along the border of the heels. In very dry skin secondary fissuring may occur, particularly along the medial border of the heel. Occasionally, callus formation may occur along the sulci of the nail edge (onychophosis) giving rise to pain on compression of the affected nail.

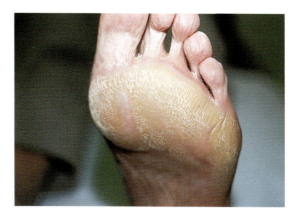

Figure 3.5
Superficial callus formation across metatarsal heads.

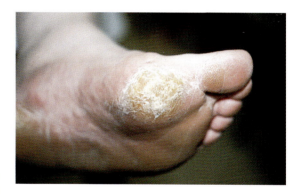

Figure 3.6
Callus under first metatarsal head.

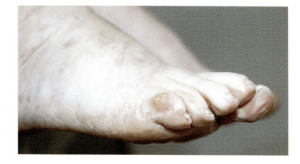

Figure 3.7
Lateral callus on fifth toe, due to inadequate footwear.

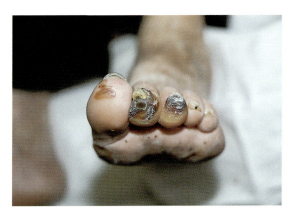

Figure 3.8
Heavy callus development on the toes with bleeding into the lesion (may lead to ulceration).

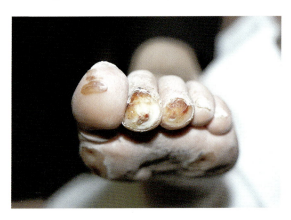

Figure 3.9
Same toe as in Figure 3.8 after debridement.

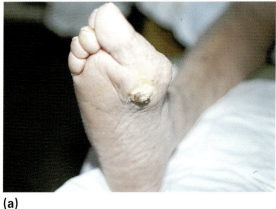

(a)

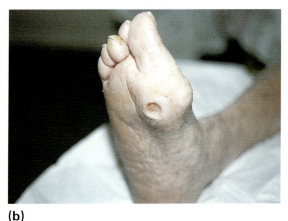

(b)

Figure 3.10
(a) Large plantar corn.
(b) After enucleation.

Corns (clavus)

This is considered to be a later stage from callosity (Figures 3.10–3.14). Essentially it is a more circumscribed lesion which is moulded into a central nucleus at the area of highest pressure, often at sites of skin located over bony prominences, e.g. dorsal interphalangeal joints, etc. The conical nucleus projects downwards into the dermis, causing more pain than callosities. Corns can be found on any area of the foot but most commonly occur on the dorsum and apices of the digits, across the plantar surface under the metatarsal heads and heel areas. Occasionally they are found in between the toes; various types of corn exist.

Hard corn (heloma durum). This is the most common type of corn, which as the name suggests is hard and dry (Figure 3.11). It is located predominantly on and in between the digits and under the metatarsal heads and the

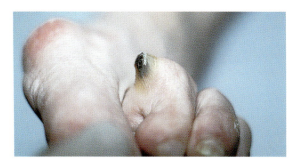

Figure 3.11
Hard corn interdigitally, due to pressure from hallux valgus deformity.

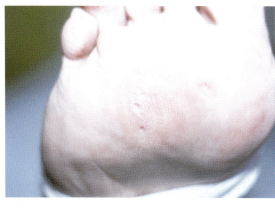

(a)

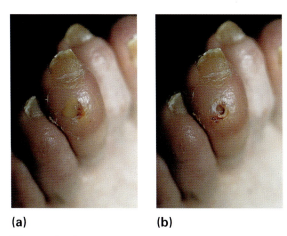

(a)   **(b)**

Figure 3.12

(a) (Painless) infected corn in a diabetic.
(b) After enucleation.

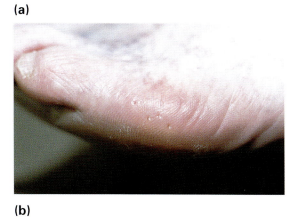

(b)

Figure 3.14
(a, b) Seed corns.

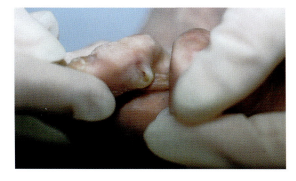

Figure 3.13
Soft corn.

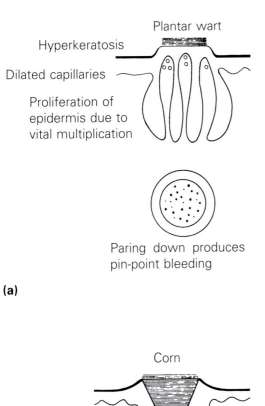

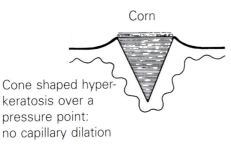

(a)

(b)

Figure 3.15

(a) Paring down a plantar wart produces pinpoint bleeding.
(b) Paring down a corn produces a decreasing cone of keratin.

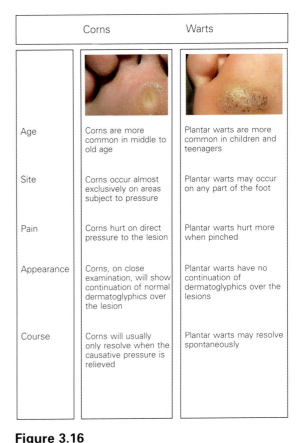

	Corns	Warts
Age	Corns are more common in middle to old age	Plantar warts are more common in children and teenagers
Site	Corns occur almost exclusively on areas subject to pressure	Plantar warts may occur on any part of the foot
Pain	Corns hurt on direct pressure to the lesion	Plantar warts hurt more when pinched
Appearance	Corns, on close examination, will show continuation of normal dermatoglyphics over the lesion	Plantar warts have no continuation of dermatoglyphics over the lesions
Course	Corns will usually only resolve when the causative pressure is relieved	Plantar warts may resolve spontaneously

Figure 3.16

Differential diagnosis between a corn and a verruca (plantar wart).

heel. Other types of corns are considered to be variants of this lesion. The hard corn is frequently mistaken for a plantar wart. Figure 3.15 shows the structural difference diagrammatically. Figure 3.16 highlights the main points of differential diagnosis.

Soft corn (heloma molle). These lesions are found exclusively in the inter-digital spaces, most commonly between the fourth and fifth toe (Figure 3.17). The major change is a white, macerated raised lesion (3–9 mm in size) with a 'rubbery' texture. Maceration occurs due to sweat accumulation in between adjacent toes.

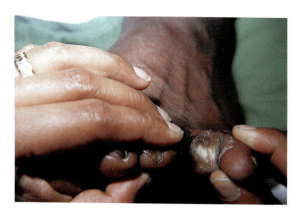

Figure 3.17

Soft corn between fourth and fifth toes.

In comparison with hard corns these lesions tend to be much more painful, particularly when the toes are compressed laterally. Soft corns usually develop where two hard surfaces oppose each other, i.e. around the inter-phalangeal joints of the toes, with the skin trapped in between. As a result 'kissing' lesions may be observed. Chronic maceration inter-digitally compromises the epidermis and may subsequently lead to secondary bacterial or fungal infection of the lesion.

Assessment of digital shape, foot function and footwear is important to elucidate the cause of soft corns. Occlusive footwear together with tight fitting hosiery can provide occlusive conditions and high inter-digital pressures.

Seed corns (heloma milliare). These lesions, of unknown aetiology, are so called because of their 'millet seed' appearance in the epidermis (Figure 3.14). Their distribution can be anywhere on the sole of the foot, also occasionally affecting the non-weight-bearing areas of the arch and dorsum, suggesting that these lesions are not always caused by pressure.

Unlike hard lesions seed corns have little overlying callus and may appear singularly or in small clusters. They are seen particularly on hypohidrotic skin.

Fibrous or intractable plantar keratoma (IPK). The above terms are often used to describe long standing corns which do not respond to normal conservative treatments. Clinically, these are very pronounced and have a white macerated appearance at their borders (Figure 3.18). The underlying dermis may show localized fibrotic changes, an adaptation to prolonged pressure.

Complication of callosity/corn formation

If the forces causing hyperkeratosis are not treated (Figures 3.19, 3.20) the lesion may become more hyperkeratotic within limits. When pressure exceeds that sustainable by the skin, ulceration can occur. This may or may not be preceded by haemorrhage into the lesion. This infiltrates the lesion from the dermal level; clinically it may appear as reddish-brown or black specks visible within the lesion. Unless the force is reduced or resolved ulceration will

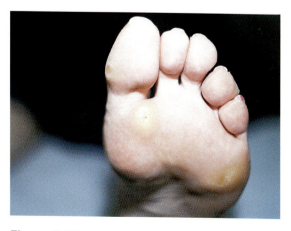

Figure 3.18

Fibrous or intractable plantar keratoma (IPK).

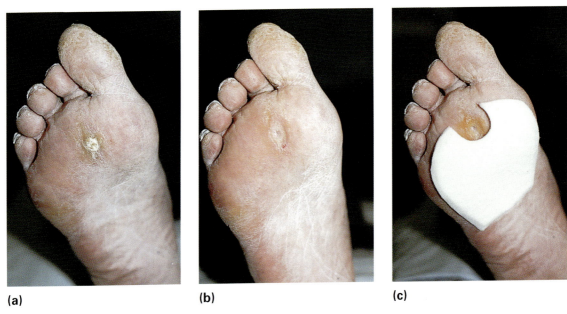

(a)   (b)   (c)

Figure 3.19

(a) Plantar corn.
(b) After enucleation.
(c) Temporary felt insert to avoid pressure.

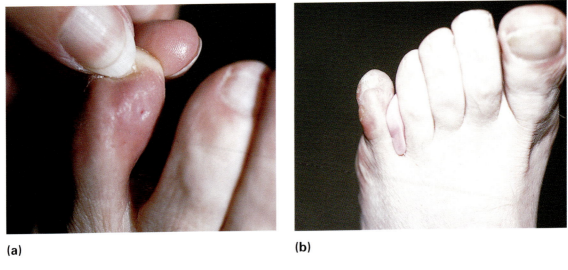

(a)   (b)

Figure 3.20

(a) Interdigital corn.
(b) Silicone spacers in place to reduce pressure between toes.

follow. Such lesions, because of their colour and appearance, occasionally mimic melanoma. Differential diagnosis is normally achieved by accurate history taking.

Palmar-plantar keratoderma (PPK)

This general term is used to encompass a wide range of rare disorders which causes excessive thickening of the stratum corneum, predominantly affecting the palms and soles. Palmar and plantar hyperkeratosis may be the only sign of the disease or it may form a single part of a widespread condition. When reporting cases of PPK, authors have traditionally used nomenclature related to appearance, distribution or histological features. This has led to a wealth of terms describing often very similar disorders.

They may be divided into:

- diffuse PPK
- focal PPK
- punctate PPK
- palmo-plantar ectodermal dysplasias.

Only the commonest or clinically distinct types are covered here. Table 3.2 gives a wider summary of the various PPKs (adapted from the classification of Stevens et al, 1996).

Table 3.2 Classification of primary palmo-plantar keratodermas (adapted from Stevens HP et al. Linkage of an American pedigree with palmo-plantar keratoderma and malignancy. *Arch Dermatol* 1996; 132: 640–51).

Diffuse palmo-plantar keratodermas
Acquired diffuse

Type I	Epidermolytic PPK
	Vurners PPK
Type II	Unna thost
	Tylosis
	Keratosis palmo-plantaris diffusa circumscripta
	Greither PPK
	Keratosis extremitatum progrediens
Type III	Erythrokeratoderma variabilis (EKV)
	Progressive symmetrical erythrokeratoderma
	Keratosis palmo-plantaris transgrediens et progrediens

Focal palmo-plantar keratodermas
Acquired focal

Type I	Striate keratoderma
	Brünauer–Fuhs–Siemens type
	Keratosis palmo-plantaris varians
	Wachters PPK
	Acral keratoderma

(Continued)

Table 3.2 *(Continued).*

Punctate palmo-plantar keratodermas	
Arsenical keratosis	
Idiopathic punctate PPK	
Idiopathic filiform porokeratotic PPK	
Type I	Buschke–Fischer–Brauer disease
	Punctata
	Keratosis papulosa
	Papulotranslucent porokeratoderma
	Keratoderma punctatum and maculosa disseminata
	Davis-Colley disease
Type II	Porokeratosis punctata palmaris and plantaris
	Punctate keratoderma
	Punctate porokeratosis of the palms and soles
	Spiny keratoderma
Type III	Focal acral hyperkeratosis
	Acrokeratoelastoidosis lichenoides
	Degenerative collagenous plaques of the hands
Palmo-plantar ectodermal dysplasias	
Type I	Focal palmo-plantar keratoderma with oral hyperkeratosis
	Keratosis palmo-plantaris nummularis
	Hereditary painful collosities
	Keratosis follicularis
	Jadassohn–Lewandowsky syndrome
	Pachyonychia congenita (type I)
Type II	Pachyonychia congenita (type II)
	Jackson–Sertoli syndrome
	Jackson–Lawler pachyonychia congenita
Type III	Tylosis
Type IV	Papillon–Lefèvre syndrome
Type V	Tyrosinaemia type II
	Oculocutaneous tyrosinaemia
	Richner–Hanhart syndrome
Type VI	Mutilating PPK with perioral hyperkeratosis
	Olmsted syndrome
Type VII	Vohwinkels syndrome
	Keratoma hereditara mutilans
Type VIII	Mal de meleda
	Acral keratoderma
Type IX	PPK with sclerodactyly
	Huriez syndrome
	Sclerotylosis
Type X	Hidrotic ectodermal dysplasia
	Fischer–Jacobsen–Clouston syndrome
	Alopecia congenita with keratosis palmo-plantaris

(Continued)

Table 3.2 *(Continued).*

	Keratosis palmaris with clubbing
Type XI	Naegeli–Franceschetti–Jadasschn syndrome
Type XII	Hyperkeratosis hyperpigmentation syndrome
Type XIII	Dermatopathia pigmentosa reticularis
Type XIV	PPK/Woolly hair/endomyocardial fibrodysplasia
Type XV	Bart–Pumphrey syndrome
	PPK and sensorineural deafness
Type XVI	Ichthyosiform erythroderma
	KID syndrome
	Desmons syndrome
Type XVII	Corneodermatosseous syndrome
Type XVIII	Charcot–Marie–Tooth with PPK/nail dystrophy
	PPK and spastic paraplegia
Type XIX	Schöpf–Schulz–Passarge syndrome

Diffuse palmo-plantar keratoderma (Figure 3.21)

Acquired diffuse PPK. Of unknown origin, this disorder produces diffuse thickening of the palms and soles. Some cases are reported to be associated with internal malignancy and rarely around the menopausal age.

Epidermolytic PPK. This has an autosomal dominant mode of inheritance, developing in the first years of life. It is limited purely to the palmar and plantar surfaces. Blistering may occur around the lesions.

Diffuse PPK (Unna Thost syndrome/tylosis). This a disorder with an autosomal dominant trait, appearing in the first few months of life. Characteristically the hyperkeratosis forms a thick, yellow blanket at the heel and gradually spreads across the plantar surface. Palmar involvement occurs at a later stage. The dorsum of the foot and extensor surfaces are also involved.

Progressive PPK (Greithers disease). A progressive, autosomal dominant condition accompanied by hyperhidrosis. Spread may occur to the extensor surfaces of the knees, hands and elbows.

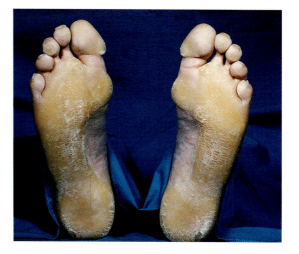

Figure 3.21
Diffuse palmo-plantar keratoderma.

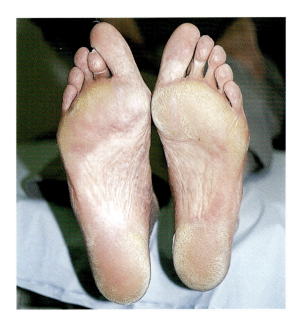

Figure 3.22
Focal PPK.

Focal palmo-plantar keratoderma
(Figure 3.22)

Striate keratoderma. A variable autosomal dominant condition which begins in infancy as palmo-plantar erythema and progresses to linear hyperkeratotic lesions. Nail changes and woolly hair may rarely be associated.

Punctate palmo-plantar keratoderma

Punctate keratoderma (keratosis punctae). This term describes a group of conditions, predominantly acquired or with an autosomal dominant mode of inheritance, which show areas of punctate hyperkeratosis across the palms and soles. These vary in appearance and may be filiform (spine like), craterform, corn like or pinhead-sized keratotic papules. Most

frequently the condition only develops after puberty. Various forms of the disease (particularly late onset) have been associated with internal malignancy.

Arsenical ingestion. Given as 'tonics' many decades ago or for the treatment of skin diseases (e.g. psoriasis), arsenic produces small brown keratoses on the palms and soles.

Palmo-plantar ectodermal dysplasias

These conditions show PPK and encompass other ectodermal defects (hair/tooth/nail/neurological signs).

Papillon–Lefèvre syndrome. An autosomal recessive disorder characterized by the early development (1–5 years of age) of PPK accompanied by erythema and hyperhidrosis. Lesions may also be present on the knees and elbows. Other abnormalities which accompany the disorder include gingivitis (causing premature tooth loss), intra-cranial calcification, recurrent skin infections, arachnodactyly and onychogryphosis.

Pachyonycia congenita. Besides PPK (in 60 per cent of cases) this autosomal dominant condition exhibits nail thickening, hyperhidrosis and leucokeratosis affecting the mucous membranes (Figure 3.23).

Vohwinkel syndrome (mutilating keratoderma). An autosomal dominant trait beginning as a diffuse honeycomb PPK in infancy and associated with alopecia of the scalp, hearing loss, myopathy and blistering of the soles of the feet. The condition continues into later life with the development of constrictive fibrous bands around the digits which may lead to auto-amputation by 'chronic gangrene'.

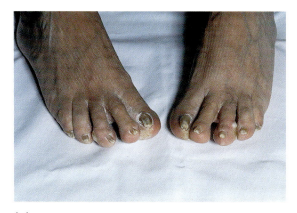

(a)

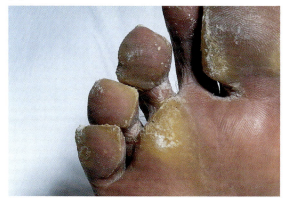

(b)

Figure 3.23

(a) Nail changes in pachyonychia congenita.
(b) Skin involvement in pachonychia congenita.

Olmsted syndrome (congenital palmo-plantar and perioral keratoderma). An extremely rare condition, characterized by PPK and perioral hyperkeratotic plaques. Other ectodermal defects may be present.

Occulo-cutaneous tyrosinaemia (Richner Hanhart syndrome). Transmitted as an autosomal recessive condition, the disorder typically develops in the first two years of life. Plantar erythema precedes hyperkeratosis of the soles. Early lesions appear as pinpoint keratoses

which gradually increase in size to form larger punctate lesions. Eye disease such as hyperlacrimation, photophobia and corneal ulceration may lead to blindness.

Mal de meleda. This is a rare disorder with both autosomal dominant and recessive patterns of inheritance, developing in the first two years of life, initially as palmo-plantar erythema. The keratoderma is not restricted to the palms and soles, spreading onto the knees, elbows and dorsal surfaces of the hands and feet. Nail changes reported include koilonychia and onychogryphosis.

Howel–Evans–Clarke syndrome. A rare autosomal dominant PPK of late onset characterized by the development of squamous cell carcinoma of the oesophagus in 70 per cent of sufferers by the age of 65.

Other causes of hyperkeratosis affecting the foot

Some acquired disorders, particularly dermatological diseases may cause hyperkeratosis of the foot: These are discussed in the appropriate sections elsewhere in the book:

- **psoriasis** (see page 91)
- **eczema/dermatitis** (see page 98)
- **lichen planus** – is a variable cause. The commonest pattern is an acute eruption of itchy papules.

Lichen planus

Sites of predilection: wrists, ankles and the small of the back; lichen planus may affect the mouth and genitalia.

Clinical features include:

- Skin lesions: (a) flat-topped; (b) shiny; (c) polygonal
- Surface — fine network of dots or lines called 'Wickham's striae'
- Colour — 'violaceous' (reddish-purple).
- Oral — lacy, reticulate streaks on the cheeks, gums and lips

In the majority of patients, the eruption settles over a period of a few months. There are a number of variants, some of which are more persistent:

- Hypertrophic, lichenified lumps appear on the legs and dorsum of the feet (Figure 3.24)
- Atrophic: largely seen in the mouth, lesions may be very chronic; small risk of carcinoma
- Follicular: may result in permanent scarring and hair loss
- Nail disease: nail changes may be very slight, or may lead to complete nail loss
- Drug induced
- Apart from the nail changes, the disease may present on the foot as (often painful) hyperkeratosis or painful progressive erosions

Aetiology: lichen planus appears to be a T-cell-mediated attack on the epidermal cells, predominantly at the dermo-epidermal junction. Similar changes are seen in the graft-versus-host reactions after bone marrow transplantation. However, the cause of lichen planus in most instances remains unknown. Topical steroids may give some relief; severe forms may require systemic steroids, oral retinoids or immunosuppressive agents.

- *Lymphoedematous keratoderma* — chronic lymphoedema on the lower limbs may cause prominent creasing and thickening of the skin on the dorsum of the foot. Chronic changes include fibrosis and papillomatous, wart-like projections. Dark brown areas of hyperkeratosis may appear, which are very adherent. Chronic lymphatic distension around the heel may lead to hyperkeratosis and fissuring along the borders of the foot. Secondary

mechanical hyperkeratosis may occur if the oedema causes footwear to be too tight
- *Keratoderma climatericum* — this is an idiopathic disorder that primarily affects obese women around the age of 45–50. Initially erythema and then reddish brown hyperkeratotic papules develop on the weight-bearing areas of the feet mainly around the heels and metatarsal heads. Painful fissuring may follow together with similar palmar involvement
- *Reiters disease* — keratoderma blennhorragica is a rare manifestation of this disease. It presents as an erythematous, hyperkeratotic eruption of the palms and soles. Similar changes to pustular psoriasis may be present

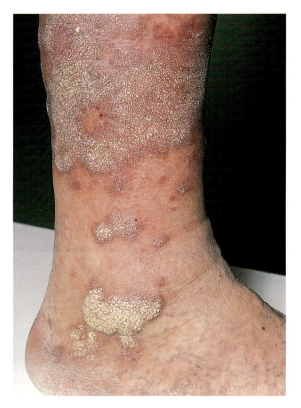

Figure 3.24

Hypertrophic (hyperkeratotic) lichen planus.

although pustulation is not a constant feature. This type is associated with HLA B27: arthropathic changes are often present

- *Hypothyroidism* — hyperkeratosis of the palms and soles may be one sign of this. It rapidly subsides with appropriate treatment of the underlying condition
- *Pityriasis rubra pilaris* — as part of this disorder, a uniform thickening of the soles may occur interrupted by 'islands' of normal skin. The hyperkeratosis is often accompanied by erythema, fissuring and peeling of the epidermis. Follicular hyperkeratotic lesions may be seen on the dorsum of the toes
- *Keratosis follicularis (Darier's disease)* — punctate keratosis and pitting is a feature of this disease. These are very subtle and may not be evident to the patient
- *Syphilis* — secondary syphilis causes pale pink macules on the soles (and palms) which rarely develop into hyperkeratotic, copper-coloured papules.

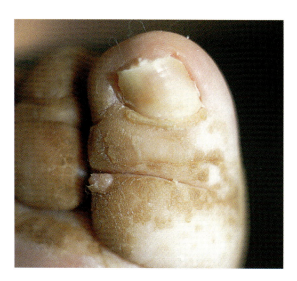

Figure 3.25
'Lymphatic' hyperkeratosis: toes.

Management of hyperkeratosis

This can range from simple measures to prevent further deterioration and symptomatic relief, to specific treatments addressing various aspects of the pathogenesis. In palmoplantar keratoderma treatment should be aimed primarily at symptomatic relief. Causes of mechanical lesions (i.e. corns and callosity) are often multifactorial; therefore various treatment modalities may be combined:

- Mechanical debridement/reduction of the lesion with a scalpel. Patients may be encouraged to assist with the regular use of callous files/pumice stones
- Use of keratolytics and caustics, i.e. salicyclic acid (up to 60 per cent), silver nitrate sticks. The use of such agents requires close supervision to avoid damage to the surrounding normal skin, particularly

in patients with reduced circulation and diabetes mellitus
- The regular use of an emollient may improve skin hydration and quality so retarding hyperkeratotic return. Emollients may also be combined with a mild keratolytic to enhance their effect and minimize fissuring potential
- The use of pressure relieving devices such as small silicon toe props to realign or protect digital deformities and simple felt padding as short term pressure relief.

Footwear adjustment and orthoses

When poor foot function is suspected, a full biomechanical assessment may highlight the need for custom-made insoles or orthoses, either to realign the foot or redistribute pressure away from painful lesions. This often goes hand in hand with footwear advice to the patient. In most cases mechanical hyperkeratotic lesions are the result of inappropriate footwear. Desirable features in a shoe include:

- extra depth right up to the end of the toe box
- extra width
- thick and flexible cushioning soles
- laces to hold the foot securely in the shoe and prevent shear
- seamless toe box with no internal stitching.

Pharmacological management

In widespread PPK and keratosis follicularis the use of vitamin A derivatives (retinoids) may help in retarding the development of hyperkeratotic areas (e.g. oral acetretin). They reduce epidermal cell adhesion, by interfering with desmosome development, and thus have a keratolytic effect.

Surgical management

This is only considered when all other treatment modalities have failed. With recalcitrant punctate areas of hyperkeratosis or IPKs electrosurgery has been used; however, scarring is a risk and unless the cause is eradicated recurrence is likely.

Where lesions develop over bony prominences, excision or shaving of bone may prove beneficial. Digital deformity may also be amenable to minor surgery. Careful planning is required to prevent drastic alterations in load bearing patterns and subsequent counter lesions at other new pressure or friction sites.

ULCERATION

Being at the end of the circulatory and neurological 'trees' the foot is particularly vulnerable to disease of both vascular and neurological systems. The foot is also subject to trauma from ground reaction forces and footwear. These factors often combine to produce ulceration. Infection may complicate these lesions resulting in osteomyelitis and/or gangrene often necessitating amputation.

Ulcers arise where loss of viability of skin tissue results in exposure of dermal and/or sub-dermal tissue. Ulcers arise as a result of various causes. In general, the principal process is one of tissue ischaemia. Ischaemia causes skin necrosis with resultant ulceration. Various factors are responsible for causing ischaemia of the foot, these include:

- neuropathy
- atherosclerosis
- microangiopathy (arteriolosclerosis)
- trauma
- venous stasis
- anaemia
- infection.

In many cases, several factors co-exist placing a foot at increased risk of ulceration. Ulcers of the foot are generally classed according to cause. Table 3.3 lists the various types of ulcer affecting the lower limb and their characteristics.

Infection

All ulcers are susceptible to secondary infection. In practice it is often difficult to judge between commensal 'non-pathogenic' organisms and causative ones. Infection of neuropathic, venous and decubitus ulcers is likely to involve both aerobic and anaerobic organisms. Infection in deep lesions has a tendency to rapid spread and may lead to penetration of the ulcer to involve periosteum and bone. Resulting osteomyelitis will result in sequestration and chronicity. Osteomyelitis complicating an ulcer often requires excision, amputation or long-term antibiotic therapy. Any ulcer on the foot of more than a few weeks duration should be X-rayed particularly in diabetic subjects.

Infection of ischaemic ulcers commonly involves anaerobic organisms. Cellulitis and rapid spread of infection is likely in patients with compromised immunity or severe ischaemia. Oral antibiotics are often unable to reach the site of infection at the level of the ulcer. In these cases topical anti-anaerobic antibiotics (e.g. metronidazole) are often successful. This is probably the only indication for the use of topical antibiotics in the management of foot ulcers.

Spread of infection as a result of foot ulcers may involve the following:

- cellulitis: infection of connective tissue (red, hot and swollen foot)
- lymphangitis: infection of lymph vessels (red streaks up the leg — lymphangitis)
- lymphadenitis: infection of lymph nodes (hot, tender, palpable nodes)
- bacteraemia: presence of bacteria in the blood stream (constitutional signs)

Table 3.3 Classification of foot ulcers and their characteristic clinical features.

Ulcer Type	Characteristic features
Neuropathic ulcer (Figures 3.26–3.31)	Painless ulceration Typically affect weight-bearing areas Deep ulcers common Hyperkeratosed edges Red base of wound Highly exudative and sloughy Irregular edges/borders Pulses present, skin quality good Surrounding skin may be macerated
Ischaemic ulcer (Figure 3.32a–c)	Punched out appearance Often painful Usually shallow Dry base of wound No hyperkeratosis to edges of border Little exudate or slough Usually affect extremities (toes and heel) lack of pulses Surrounding skin dry and atrophic
Decubitus ulcer (pressure sore) (Figures 3.33, 3.34)	Often deep Occur at sites of excess or prolonged pressure (e.g. heel, inter-digital) Painful (unless co-existing neuropathy) Inflamed, 'shiny', surrounding skin Edges not hyperkeratosed Sloughy and exudative Surrounding skin may be macerated/blister Generally round or oval shaped

(Continued)

Table 3.3 *(Continued)*

Venous (syn varicose, stasis) ulcer (Figure 3.35)	Occur at ankle/malleolar level Large, shallow lesions Associated venous stasis eczema and oedema Haemosiderosis (pigmentation) of skin Highly sloughy and exudative Well demarcated edges
Fungating ulcer (malignant/neoplastic)	Unusual changes in longstanding lesion Rolled edges Poorly demarcated border Hypergranulation evident Foul smelling Highly exudative (sero-purulent discharge) May be constitutional symptoms (anorexia, weight-loss, diarrhoea etc.)
Mixed aetiology ulcers (Figure 3.36) usually ischaemic/neuropathic – can be venous/ischaemic – decubitus/neuropathic	Features of these ulcers are dependent on the dominant aetiologies (see above) Mixed aetiology ulcers are extremely common, especially amongst diabetic patients, rheumatoids and the elderly

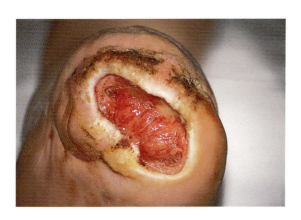

Figure 3.26
Neuropathic ulcer across the metatarsals following amputation of the toes.

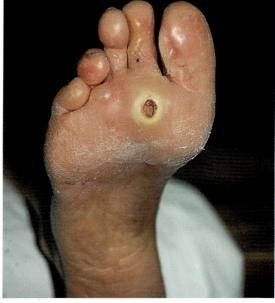

Figure 3.27
Neuropathic ulcer over prominent second metatarsal head.

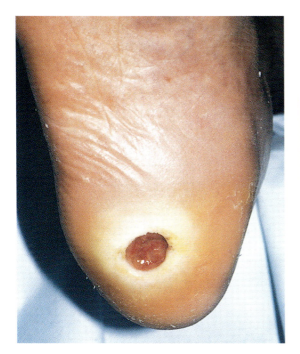

Figure 3.28
Neuropathic ulcer following puncture wound.

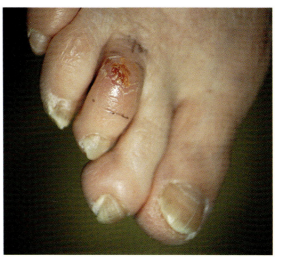

Figure 3.30
Neuropathic ulcer on toe, due to rubbing from
footwear.

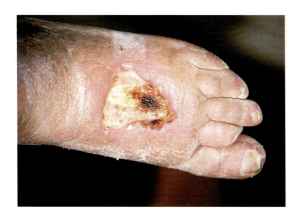

Figure 3.29
Neuropathic ulcer, due to pressure from a zip
fastener on a slipper.

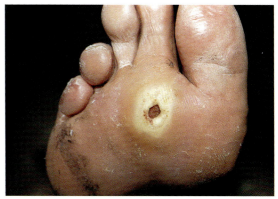

Figure 3.31
Neuropathic ulcer, due to pressure over
metatarsal head.

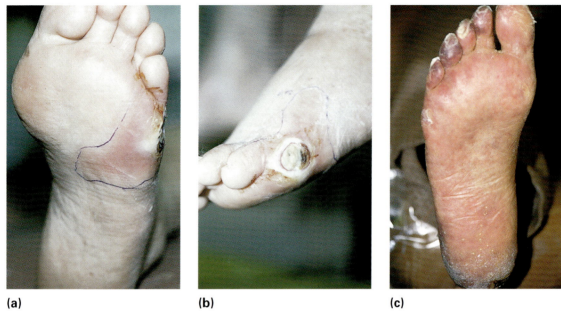

(a)   (b)   (c)

Figure 3.32
(a–c) Ischaemic ulcers.

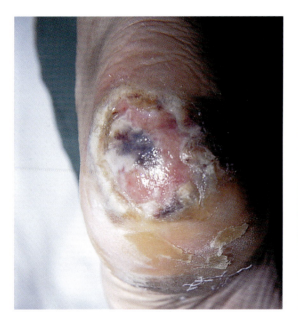

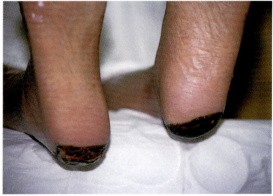

Figure 3.33
A shallow pressure sore on the heel of a diabetic.

Figure 3.34
Pressure sore on heels, due to prolonged bed rest.

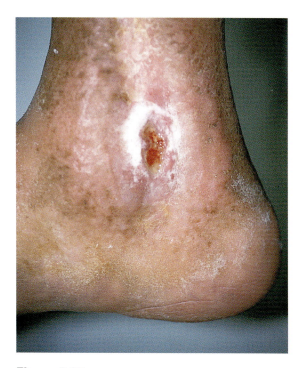

Figure 3.35
Venous leg ulcer adjacent to the medial malleolus.

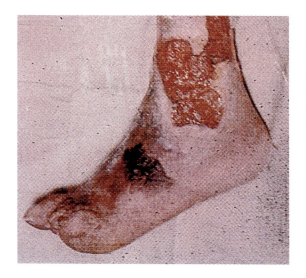

Figure 3.36
Ulceration due to venous and arterial/arteriolar occlusion.

- septicaemia: presence of multiplying bacteria in the bloodstream (pyrexia)
- toxaemia: presence of bacterial toxins in the bloodstream (pyrexia, coma, death).

Patients at increased risk of infection are those with compromised immunity. Table 3.4 lists conditions in which patient's immunity is likely to be compromised.

Table 3.4 Factors associated with compromised immunity.

Diabetes mellitus
Human immunodeficiency virus infection
Infectious mononucleosis infection
Cytomegalovirus infection
Malnutrition
Cushing's syndrome/disease
Long term systemic corticosteroid therapy
Immuno-suppressive drugs
Leukaemia
Lymphomas
Old age
Genetic disorders (DiGeorge syndrome, etc.)

Gangrene

Gangrene is defined as necrosis of tissue with digestion by saprophytic bacteria. The foot is the commonest site of gangrene, with the toes and heel being particularly vulnerable in susceptible individuals (Figure 3.37). Gangrene may arise as a result of direct primary local trauma or infection, or more usually occur secondary to some other underlying pathology. There are three main types of gangrene:

- gas gangrene
- dry gangrene
- moist gangrene.

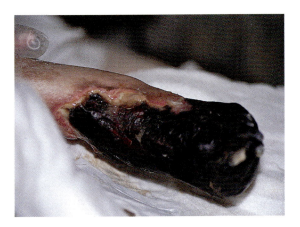

Figure 3.37
Acute arterial occlusion with extensive tissue necrosis.

Gas gangrene

Gas gangrene is a primary form of gangrene with a specific aetiology. It is caused by infection with *clostridium welchi*, a micro-organism present in soil. Gas gangrene may occur following a severe crushing injury or following penetrating trauma resulting in much loss of tissue. Cellulitis is evident with gas crepitus present in over 80 per cent of cases. Pronounced oedema and deep red discolouration of the affected part is evident. A foul smelling, serous, brown exudate is produced. Spread may be rapid, to involve muscle and bone. The gangrene is usually well demarcated. However, spread of infection from cellulitis to myositis to shock, toxic delirium and death can occur from one to several days. Prompt diagnosis and treatment is essential. Diagnosis is assisted by culture and X-rays. Radiographs may show local gas production. Treatment requires wound debridement and intra-venous penicillin G, or tetracycline. Sometimes amputation of the affected part is required to control spread of infection.

Dry gangrene

This is the most common form of gangrene affecting the feet. Dry gangrene arises as a result of progressive ischaemia and tissue necrosis. Affected tissues become 'mummified' (Figure 3.38). Tissue appears shrunken, dark in colour and is well demarcated from surrounding healthy tissue. Dry gangrene commonly affects tissues supplied by diseased end-arteries (e.g. digits, heel, lateral and medial borders of forefoot). Underlying macro-vascular and/or micro-vascular disease is usually pronounced. Dry gangrene can be extremely painful in non-neuropathic individuals. In these cases amputation is often necessary to relieve pain and prevent secondary infection. In many patients, however, this type is a painless process owing to co-existing sensory neuropathy. In these cases, surgical amputation is not often necessary. The affected part will usually slough off (auto-amputation). Long-term prophylactic antibiotics may be necessary to prevent spread of infection.

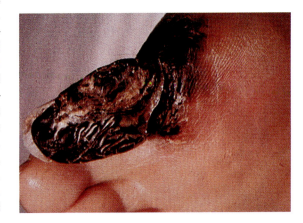

Figure 3.38
Dry gangrene of the hallux.

Moist gangrene

Moist gangrene occurs where there is purulent infection related to ischaemia. It may occur alongside or in tissue adjacent to an area affected by dry gangrene. In the foot, moist gangrene presents as a grossly oedematous foot with poorly demarcated cellulitis and necrosis. Moist gangrene is often associated with mixed ischaemic/venous aetiologies and long-term venous stasis in a patient with peripheral vascular disease. Spread of infection to involve bone and systemic spread is common if the infection is not promptly treated. Radical wound debridement, intravenous antibiotics and/or amputation is often required.

Patients at risk of foot ulcers

Various groups of patients are at increased risk of developing foot ulcers. These groups are primarily those with one or more of the following risk factors:

- immuno-deficiency
- angiopathy or microangiopathy
- neuropathy (motor, sensory and/or autonomic)
- lower limb venous disease
- inflammatory arthropathy (e.g. rheumatoid arthritis)
- foot deformity.

Some systemic diseases, including diabetes mellitus, are complicated by one or more of the above factors. Such patients are therefore classed 'at risk' of foot ulceration, infection, gangrene and amputation.

Foot ulcers in diabetes mellitus

Chronically high blood glucose levels (>10 mmol^{-1}) may be associated with pathological changes to peripheral nerves and vessels. Resultant neuropathy and vascular disease is associated with loss of tissue viability in affected individuals. The key to diabetic ulcer prevention lies with good control of blood glucose levels and early detection of pathology followed by appropriate therapy and advice.

Diabetic neuropathy is typically symmetrical and involves sensory, motor and autonomic peripheral nerves (distal symmetrical polyneuropathy). Assessment of diabetic neuropathy should attempt to investigate function of peripheral nerves, and highlight any effects of peripheral nerve damage. Sensory nerve assessment involves tests of perception at various sites of the foot including: light touch using mono-filaments, heat and cold perception, vibration using a tuning fork or neurothesiometer and pain perception. Sensory mapping of the foot can then indicate areas of impaired sensation at risk of undetected trauma and ulceration.

Early signs of sensory neuropathy in the diabetic foot are often related to increases in plantar pressure. The plantar skin responds to plantar pressure initially by hypertrophy. In the early stages this is evidenced by enhanced dermatoglyphics at the site of excess pressure. Such areas should be given priority attention as these sites are at high risk of ulceration. Hyperkeratosis (corns and callus) is also indicative of high pressure and indicates risk of ulceration. A neuropathic patient may not complain of pain in corns or calluses of the feet and many lesions are ignored or neglected. The presence of hyperkeratosis in a diabetic should always be viewed with suspicion and the lesion and the underlying pressure managed appropriately.

Early ulcerative damage is indicated by extravasation of hyperkeratosis, inflammation of surrounding skin, or exudation. In these cases the patient and health professional may wrongly judge that the foot is unaffected as the skin may still be intact and no obvious signs of ulceration may be apparent. In fact, chiropodists and podiatrists debriding complicated hyperkeratotic lesions are often blamed for the resulting exposed ulcer.

Motor neuropathy affecting the foot in a diabetic patient can result in intrinsic muscle weakness and foot deformity. Typical deformities affect the digits, resulting in retraction of the toes. Retracted toes are often related to plantarflexion of the associated metatarsals. This deformity creates areas vulnerable to pressure at the metatarsal heads, apices of the toes and the prominent dorsal inter-phalangeal joints. This is worsened by distal shifting of the protective fibro-fatty padding normally located between the metatarsal heads and the plantar skin.

Autonomic neuropathy in the foot affects the quality of the skin. Normal sympathetic tone to the foot ensures that sweat and sebaceous secretions are produced to maintain normal skin hydration and normal skin pH. In autonomic neuropathy hydration and pH of the skin changes results in dryness of the skin and loss of antibacterial 'acid mantle'. Dry skin is less able to adapt to changes in pressure, shear or friction. The skin therefore becomes less resistant to trauma; it is also more likely to dry, crack and fissure. These fissures may bleed, ulcerate and become infected. Loss of the acid mantle increases the risk of colonization by pathogenic organisms and subsequent wound infection. Autonomic neuropathy also has a role to play in the pathology of the Charcot foot (neuroarthropathy) characterized by gross deformity of the tarsal joints. Autonomic neuropathy increases flow of blood into the tarsus resulting in this gross osseous change, usually seen in association with mild injury.

Diabetic polyneuropathy can therefore result in gross bony deformity of the tarsal joints producing a 'rocker bottom' Charcot foot (Figure 3.39). Normal shock absorption and propulsion is lost in the Charcot foot, which results in the development of plantar foci of abnormally high pressure. These pressure areas are highly prone to ulceration. Digital retraction is also common as a secondary deformity of the Charcot foot. Retracted digits are at risk of ulceration where they come into contact with the ground or the upper of the shoe.

Severe pes-plano valgus deformity associated with Charcot foot types can result in areas of high pressure at the medial aspect of the ankle. Pressure from footwear may result in blistering and/or ulceration in this area.

Management of the Charcot foot can be a particular challenge. The key to success lies in effective pressure redistribution. Use of bespoke or orthopaedic/semi-orthopaedic footwear with pressure-redistributive insoles are often indicated as a preventative measure where areas of high pressure are 'pre-ulcerative'. Where plantar ulceration has already occurred, use of walking casts such as the Scotch-Cast boot is often necessary to achieve complete pressure relief from the affected area (Figure 3.40). Alternative strategies adopting Air-Casts and below knee plaster-of-Paris casts have also proven useful in some patients. Care must be taken to avoid transferring pressure to another site unable to withstand it. Pressure should therefore be transferred to as wide an area as possible, reducing the risk of transfer lesions. In severe cases of deep neuropathic ulceration, use of a wheel-chair, crutches or complete bed rest may be necessary.

Once healing has been achieved, careful assessment of plantar pressures is necessary. A variety of techniques for plantar pressure measurement are available from very simple and inexpensive methods involving ink-mats (e.g. Harris and Beath mat) to computerized transducer bases systems (e.g. Musgrave). Pressure management is often the key to preventing recurrence of ulceration in the diabetic foot. Pressure measurement can also be used to assess the efficacy of padding used to redistribute pressure from vulnerable areas.

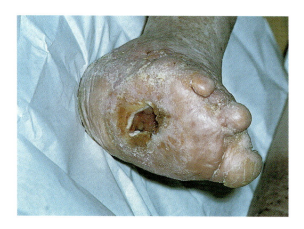

Figure 3.39

'Charcot' changes in a diabetic subject with secondary ulceration.

Peripheral vascular assessment in the diabetic patient should include assessment of both large and small vessels. Use of Doppler vasoflow is useful to determine patency of large vessels proximal to the dorsalis pedis and posterior tibial arteries. Segmental systolic pressures can help to determine the level of occlusion in large vessel disease. Comparison of ankle with brachial systolic pressures can help to indicate the severity of macroangiopathy and may help to predict the likely ability of a foot ulcer to heal. However, this test can be complicated by peripheral arterial calcification

Pressure measurement is also used to assess the effect of such padding on surrounding skin in order to prevent transfer lesions.

Vascular changes complicating diabetes mellitus may involve both large and small arteries (macroangiopathy and microangiopathy). Poorly controlled diabetics are at increased risk of atherosclerosis and medial arterial calcification. These disorders also occur more distally in diabetics than in non-diabetics, often affecting vessels distal to the popliteal fossa. This is unusual in non-diabetic patients. Such large vessel disease may compromise the blood supply to the feet and result in ischaemia. Ischaemic ulceration of the periphery is therefore a consequence of this process.

Micro-vascular disease in diabetics primarily affects the small arterioles and capillaries. Basement membrane thickening occurs which interferes with gas exchange and perfusion. Micro-thrombi may completely obliterate a small vessel causing small areas of necrosis. Micro-vascular disease will place affected tissue at increased risk of ischaemic ulceration, and the reduced oxygen availability will result in slow healing wounds.

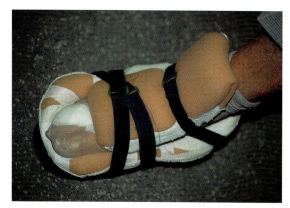

(a)

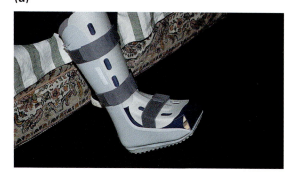

(b)

Figure 3.40

(a, b) Walking devices that can offload pressure but still allow the patient to be ambulant.

in diabetic patients. Calcification of peripheral arteries will give an abnormally high ankle systolic pressure.

Exercise stress testing is a more reliable method of assessment; measuring the ankle systolic pressure at rest and again following 2–3 minutes of light exercise. Normally, hyperaemia induced by exercise should induce an increase in ankle systolic pressure which should recover to the resting level within 2 minutes. In mild peripheral vascular disease, the post-exercise ankle systolic pressure falls below that of the resting pressure but returns to the resting level within 2 minutes. In severe peripheral arterial disease, the post-exercise ankle systolic pressure drops (often significantly or to a non-detectable level!) and takes greater than 2–3 minutes to restore to the resting level. These pressure measurements can be repeated with the sphygmomanometer cuff placed mid-way up the tibia, at the distal aspect of the thigh and at the proximal aspect of the thigh. These segmental pressure measurements and post-exercise pressure measurements are extremely useful in assessing the degree and level of macroangiopathy in diabetic patients.

Assessment of microvascular disease usually involves simple clinical methods including assessment of capillary re-filling time. More specialized tests may also be carried out. Capillaroscopy is a technique which involves examination of the capillaries at the base of the nail. Here the capillary loops run parallel to the skin rather than perpendicular to it and are easily accessible. An oil-immersion microscope can be used to image these capillaries and check for blood flow or obstruction.

Trans-cutaneous oxygen pressure monitors can be used to monitor the oxygen perfusion in the skin of the foot. The apices of the toes are often chosen for the assessment of microvascular disease in diabetic patients. Abnormally low trans-cutaneous pressures correlate with poor tissue perfusion occurring as a result of either macrovascular or micro-

vascular disease. If a patient has an adequate macrovascular supply (i.e. good ankle systolic pressure, pulses and segmental pressures) but a poor trans-cutaneous oxygen pressure reading at the periphery, then the likely site of disease is in the small vessels. Transcutaneous oxygen pressure measurements are reliable indicators of the viability of the skin and the ability of wounds to heal (Table 3.5).

Table 3.5 Trans-cutaneous oxygen measurement of the foot.

Oxygen pressure	Rate of healing
>50 mmHg	Normal
30—50 mmHg	Slow
<30 mmHg	None

Foot ulcers in rheumatoid patients

Patients with rheumatoid arthritis are particularly at risk of foot ulcers for the following reasons:

- presence of severe deformity
- alteration of plantar pressure
- effects of corticosteroids on skin and immunity
- effects of unusual complications (e.g. vasculitis, neuropathy).

Characteristic foot deformities in rheumatoid arthritis affect the toes. Severe hallux abducto valgus deformities are common in rheumatoid patients. The widening of the forefoot resulting from this deformity can be difficult to accommodate in standard shoes. Pressure from ill-fitting footwear on the medial eminence of the first metatarsal can lead to bursitis, blistering or ulceration. Secondary retraction of the lesser toes also occurs in most cases. Digital retraction and distal displacement of the plantar fibro-fatty padding increases the plantar pressure under the forefoot. Hyperkeratotic plantar and digital lesions are therefore common. The second and third plantar metatarsal areas are particularly prone to increased plantar pressure as a result of transfer of weight from a dysfunctional first ray. Formation of adventitious bursae at these sites is relatively common in rheumatoid patients.

Ulceration in rheumatoid feet usually occurs at a previous site of hyperkeratosis. Loss of tissue viability is particularly likely if the patient is receiving systemic corticosteroid therapy, as the skin quality will be reduced and healing ability decreased. Rheumatoid foot ulcers are particularly prone to infection. If left untreated, this may rapidly progress to involve joints and bone, making amputation necessary.

Principles of prevention and management of rheumatoid foot ulcers are similar to those of diabetic foot ulcers (it is essential to identify and address the cause). Abnormal pressures must be dealt with, lesions debrided, appropriate dressings and antibacterial therapy chosen, and effective advice given to the patient. In some cases surgical referral is necessary, especially where the ulcer is deep or muscle, tendon or bone are affected.

Principles of ulcer management

The aim of wound management, after addressing the cause of the lesion, is to foster ideal conditions for healing to take place. In most cases, ideal conditions for healing will include:

- warm environment
- mildly acidic environment
- moist healing environment, avoiding tissue maceration
- protection/freedom from trauma, i.e. specialist footwear, cast or rest
- protection/freedom from infection
- adequate supply of blood (oxygen and nutrients).

A plethora of wound dressing products are available for use on foot wounds. It is important to be aware of the physical properties of dressings and how they will interact with the wound prior to selection. An ideal wound dressing would foster the above environmental factors. This usually means that careful assessment of the wound is required to determine what properties are required of the dressing to promote healing. For example, a dry necrotic ischaemic wound will have difficulty healing for the following reasons:

- cold wound surface (due to lack of blood flow)
- loss of acid mantle (ischaemia-induced reduction of sebum and sweat production)
- dry environment
- necrotic tissue provides trauma to granulation tissue
- necrotic tissue encourages infection
- lack of blood supply (poor nutrient and oxygen availability).

In this example a wound dressing would be thermally insulating, slightly acidic, occlusive, and antibacterial. In practice, necrotic tissue must be removed by debridement and the blood supply improved by surgery if appropriate. An occlusive film dressing (e.g. Opsite, Biofilm) maintains a moist healing environment, and if used in conjunction with appropriate padding (e.g. Plastazote) may also thermally insulate. Assessment in this way can ensure an effective choice of wound dressing.

Properties and indications of various types of wound dressings are given in Table 3.6. Use of topical medicaments should be avoided. There is evidence to suggest that topical antiseptic agents (creams, ointments or dressings) may reduce rates of phagocytosis and re-epithelialization. Topical antibiotics may result in allergic sensitization, with the possible exception of topical metranidazole used to treat anaerobic infection of ischaemic ulcers. For prophylaxis or treatment of bacterial infection, systemic antibiotic therapy should be prescribed in preference to topical therapy, always based on bacterial swabs for microscopy, culture and 'antibacterial sensitivity' tests.

Table 3.6 Common wound dressings and their properties and indication.

Dressing type	Examples	Properties and indications
Alginate	Kaltostat Sorbsan	Highly absorbent Form a gel on contact with exudate Ideal for heavily exuding wound including neuropathic, decubitus and venous ulcers
Polyurethane Film	Opsite (film) Biofilm Tegaderm	Occlusive dressing Good to hydrate dry tissue Ideal for dry, ischaemic wounds
Foams	Lyofoam	Thermally insulating Mechanically protective Draws exudate by capillary action Useful for mildly exuding wounds Good for inter-digital ulcers and 'cold' distal foot ulcers
Hydrocolloids	Granuflex	Biological wound dressing mimicking properties of skin Encourage de-sloughing of wound Good for sloughy venous ulcers Use on mildly exudative foot wounds
Tulles	Jelonet	Contain paraffin waxes Good to hydrate heel fissures used under occlusion
Antibacterial	Inadine Bactigras	Rarely indicated as topical antiseptic agents may delay healing Useful for burns to prevent secondary infection
Non-adherent simple	Melolin Skin-tact	Simple primary dressing Not very absorbent Suitable for non-exudative or very mildly-exudative wounds Use of more absorbent dressing (e.g. Alginate) may be used in combination

ERYTHEMA AND VASCULITIS

Erythema is a cardinal sign of inflammation and therefore accompanies many inflammatory and infective skin diseases. Vasculitis and vascular disorders may result in skin changes including hypoxia, hypercapnia, ischaemia, necrosis and ulceration. Erythematous and vasculitic skin diseases are often important indicators of co-existing systemic illness or potentially serious local pathology.

Erythema

Classification of erythema is given in Table 3.7.

Infective causes of erythema

Viral, fungal or bacterial infection (Figure 3.41) can result in erythema of the foot. Common examples of erythema of the foot due to infection include:

- bacterial — paronychia
  cellulitis
  erythrasma
- fungal — tinea pedis
  candidal infection
- viral — plantar warts
  herpes simplex lesions

Management of the infection with appropriate anti-infective drugs, or local therapy (e.g. cryosurgery for warts) usually eradicates infection and cures the erythema.

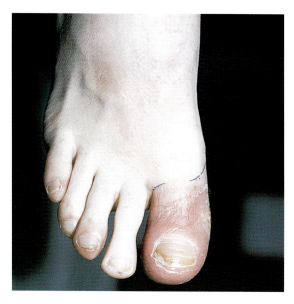

Figure 3.41
'Mixed' bacterial infection of the great toe, giving prominent erythema.

Connective tissue disorders and erythema

The principal feature of connective tissue disorders is that they cause inflammation of connective tissue. This usually leads to dermal atrophy, sclerosis or other organ defects including arthritis and pulmonary disease. Connective tissue disorders giving rise to erythema in the foot and lower limb are detailed below:

Table 3.7. Classification of erythema affecting the foot.

Class	Examples
Infection (local or systemic)	Cellulitis (bacterial)
	Herpes simplex virus
	Tinea pedis (fungal)
Connective tissue disorders	Systemic lupus erythematosus
	Scleroderma
Inflammatory	Allergic drug response
	Non-allergic drug response
	Local inflammation
Secondary erythema	Due to primary disease elsewhere, e.g. liver, endocrine, rheumatoid arthritis
	Palmar erythema

Lupus erythematosus

A range of skin patterns occur in this auto-immune disease. Some predominantly affect the skin, others affect internal organs. Lesions range from discoid lesions occurring on skin exposed sites (discoid LE) to scaly psoriasi-form plaques (subacute cutaneous LE) to periungual telangiectasia and digital erythema (systemic LE). Treatment usually includes local or systemic anti-inflammatory steroid medication or immunosuppressive agents.

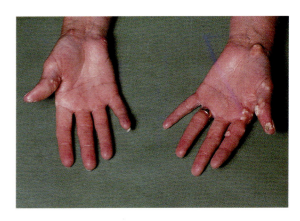

Figure 3.42
Acrosclerosis and calcification in systemic sclerosis.

Scleroderma (systemic sclerosis)

This is an idiopathic systemic condition result-ing in thickening of connective tissue and skin (Figures 3.42, 3.43). Skin becomes taut, hard and shiny. Raynaud's phenomenon and digital ischaemic ulceration with phalangeal bone resorption may occur. Treatment is difficult and unsatisfactory. Emollients are used to keep skin moist and prevent fissuring.

Sarcoidsosis

This is an idiopathic granulomatous connective tissue disorder, characterized by dermatologi-cal and systemic disease. Skin defects include erythema nodosum (Figure 3.44), patches of brownish-red papules or plaques (granulomas) and chilblains. Treatment is unsatisfactory; systemic steroids may be useful in some cases; alternatives include oral retinoids and methotrexate.

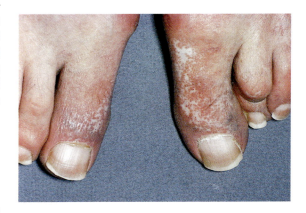

Figure 3.43
Vascular inflammation and necrosis, due to systemic sclerosis.

Inflammatory cause of erythema

As erythema is a cardinal feature of acute inflammation, it is a common finding in acute inflammatory skin conditions. Acute skin inflam-mation may result from trauma, infection, or hypersensitivity. Mechanical (pressure, shear, friction), thermal (cold, heat), or physical (radia-tion, electrical) trauma can initiate an acute inflammatory response producing erythema of the skin. Erythema thus caused is usually accompanied by other features of acute inflam-mation including pain, heat, swelling and loss of

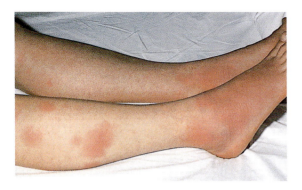

Figure 3.44
Erythema nodosum.

function. Treatment involves removing cause of trauma, RICE (rest, ice, compression, elevation) therapy and systemic anti-histamine and non-steroidal anti-inflammatory medication. Similarly, pathogenic micro-organisms initiate a host response which involves acute inflammation. Treatment of this includes appropriate anti-microbial drugs and local therapy. Allergic reactions causing erythema may occur for example due to systemic drug reactions.

Secondary causes of erythema

Erythema of skin of the foot may be seen as a secondary feature of a variety of systemic or internal diseases. Examples of factors causing secondary erythema include:

- rheumatoid arthritis
- hepatitis and cirrhosis
- malignancy
- thyroid disease
- drug use, e.g. vasodilators
- alcohol.

Secondary erythema is sometimes an important pointer to systemic illness, for example palmar erythema in liver disease. The erythema usually improves when the primary disease process or cause is treated.

Vasculitis

Vasculitis implies inflammation of blood vessels. Small and/or large vessels may be involved and the inflammation my be transient or progressive. Vasculitis disorders affecting the skin of the foot are described in Table 3.8.

Small vessel vasculitis

Acrocyanosis. This is a common peripheral circulatory defect affecting small arteries and arterioles of hands, feet, nose, ears and cheeks. Exposure to cold results in arteriolar constriction and increased blood viscosity. Oxygen availability to peripheral tissue is therefore reduced and metabolites accumulate. Skin in affected areas appears red-purple, pale or cyanotic. Slow re-warming of affected tissue

Table 3.8 Vasculitis disorders affecting the foot.

Small vessels	Large vessels
Acrocyanosis	Raynaud's phenomenon
Erythrocyanosis	Atherosclerosis
Erythema perniosis (chilblains)	Arterial embolism
Telangiectasia	Deep vein thrombosis
Erythema ab igne	Chronic venous stasis syndrome

permits restoration of normal vasomotor tone and blood viscosity. Tissues rapidly recover after a period of slow re-warming. Prevention is often the best form of management, with patients advised to wear thick, insulating clothing, including shoes and socks, and to avoid cold.

Capillaritis. A form of vasculitis affecting capillaries. The signs seen consist of large numbers of 'leaky' capillaries with subtle endothelial damage, red cell extravasation and brownish red haemosiderin 'stains'. Venous insufficiency, drugs and sometimes streptococcal infection.

Erythrocyanosis. This is a relatively common vascular disorder occurring in young typically obese women. Cold provokes a vasospastic response resulting in areas of purple-red discolouration and burning sensations over the buttocks, thighs, shins and sometimes the ankles. In severe cases, these erythrocyanotic lesions become necrotic and may be slow to heal. Avoidance of cold and use of appropriate warm clothing can help to prevent recurrence.

Perniosis (chilblains) (Figure 3.45). A familial vasospastic disorder which is often seen in the winter, producing purple-red slightly oedematous lesions of the toes, also affecting fingers and occasionally the ears and nose. Chilblains are characteristically itchy and pain is often described as 'burning'. Re-warming causes a burning sensation in lesions, especially where cold feet are re-warmed rapidly. Chilblains occur as a result of arteriolar and venular constriction triggered by cold exposure. Metabolite accumulation in sub-cutaneous tissue and hypoxia cause the skin lesions. Chilblains occasionally ulcerate and are slow to heal. Avoidance of cold, thermal insulation and in particular avoidance of rapid change from one extreme of temperature to another can help prevent chilblains. Topical and systemic vasodilators and counter irritant (rubefacients) have negligible effects.

Telangiectasia. This is the appearance of permanently dilated and visible blood vessels

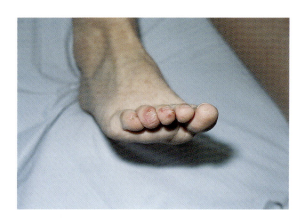

Figure 3.45
Chilblains.

(capillaries and venules) in the skin (Figure 3.46). They are seen in association with many vascular disorders and other conditions, including:

*   venous hypertension
*   liver disease (spider telangiectasia)
*   mastocytosis
*   pregnancy or oral contraception.

Telangiectasia seen on the foot is most commonly due to venous hypertension. Associated signs may include purpura and haemosiderosis. Telangiectasia is usually asymptomatic but to many patients it can be a considerable 'aesthetic' compromise. Laser therapy may successfully ablate areas with good cosmetic results.

Erythema ab igne. Common amongst patients who lack central heating and rely on open fires for warmth (Figure 3.47). It is caused by local exposure of the skin to infrared heat. Local heat exposure causes vasodilation and leakage of red cells into the skin causing haemosiderin staining, giving in conjunction with the post-inflammatory hyperpigmentation a yellow, brown colour. Scaling may occur as a result of metabolite accumulation. Advice to protect the skin from intense local heat is often all that is required to prevent worsening

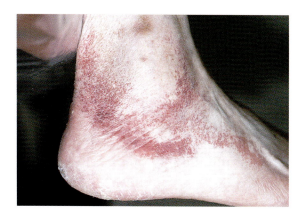

Figure 3.46
Telangiectasia.

of the disorder. It is not possible to treat existing staining.

Large vessel vasculitis

Raynaud's phenomenon. A painful and sometimes serious disorder characterized by predominantly cold-induced pallor of digits. Initially the tips of the digits are affected, becoming pale,

followed shortly by painful cyanosis; the area then develops a deep red/purple colour. Complications may involve loss of digit 'pulp' substance, ulceration and gangrene. Occasionally, digits may require amputation. Raynaud's phenomenon may be associated with SLE, scleroderma (Figure 3.48), acrosclerosis, ergotamine, peripheral neuropathy and polycythaemia. Pneumatic and/or hammer drill operators are at increased risk of the disease. Treatment requires avoidance of significant cold exposure and adequate thermal insulation. Vasodilators are rarely effective. Patients may occasionally require sympathectomy.

Atherosclerosis. The formation of atheroma in large and medium-sized arteries and is a common cause of lower limb vascular disease. Obstruction leads to signs of ischaemia. Patients may complain of exertion pain in lower limb muscles (intermittent claudication), or there may be signs of impaired perfusion of the skin of the foot. Severe atherosclerosis of the lower limb arteries often causes foot ulceration, gangrene and amputation. The effects of chronic ischaemia are discussed in the section on foot ulceration (page 48).

Arterial embolism. The obstruction of blood supply to the lower limb and foot, usually an

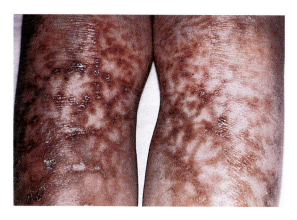

Figure 3.47
Erythema ab igne.

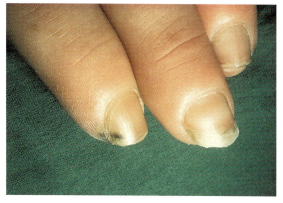

Figure 3.48
Raynaud's disease with acrosclerosis in systemic sclerosis.

acute event. Acute ischaemia occurs resulting in clinical signs of pain, paraesthesia, severe cold, absence of pulses and pallor; the foot becomes deathly pale, cold and painful. Urgent anticoagulant or surgical treatment to remove or 'dissolve' the clot is essential if the foot or limb is to be preserved.

Deep vein thrombosis. This results in restriction of venous return from the lower limb and venous hypertension distal to the site of occlusion. The skin is inevitably affected by this: in acute cases, the limb and foot becomes deep red or extremely pale in colour. Tissue hypoxia may occur secondary to the oedema that is often present. In these acute cases urgent anticoagulant treatment is essential. Long-term effects of DVT are referred to as post-thrombophlebitic syndrome or chronic venous stasis syndrome.

Chronic venous stasis syndrome. This follows acute deep vein thrombosis or other long term venous hypertension, patients may present with many associated skin signs. Telangiectasia, purpura, haemosiderosis, pitting oedema, stasis eczema, varicose veins and echymoses all occur. In severe cases, fibrin deposition leads to a 'woody hard' appearance of the leg and non-pitting oedema. Skin of the ankle area is particularly affected and vulnerable. Skin ulceration is an unfortunate common consequate of venous stasis. Treatment is to improve venous return and reduce venous pressure (exercise, compression, elevation).

INFECTIVE DISEASES

Many viral, bacterial and fungal organisms can produce primary or secondary infection of the foot and toenails; or significantly colonize existing primary pathology. It is important to recognize where organisms are indeed pathogenic and equally important not to treat those that are known commensals — to avoid false optimism regarding potential

for cure and to limit the potential for resistant strains to appear. However one must remember that in AIDS and those receiving immunosuppressive drugs even apparently banal saprophytes may become systematized. These normal flora include some staphylococci, corynebacteria, pseudomonas species and many fungi of dermatophytic, yeast and saprophytic type.

Bacterial infections

Bacterial infections that may specifically localize to the foot, or cause damage to foot function, include:

- corynebacteria
  - pitted keratolysis (synonym, keratolysis plantare sulcatum)
  - erythrasma
- streptococci
  - blistering distal dactylitis
  - erysipelas/cellulitis
- staphylococci
  - impetigo
  - acute paronychia
- tuberculosis
  - persistent ulceration
  - warty plaques
  - granulomatous lupus vulgaris plaques
- leprosy
  - skeletal and skin results of nerve damage.

Pitted keratolysis

As a result of erosion of the keratinous layer of soles of feet by corynebacterium organisms particularly around sweat pores initially, punctate erosions coalesce to give larger circular lesions (Figure 3.49). These lesions look rather hydrated and may be moist and tender

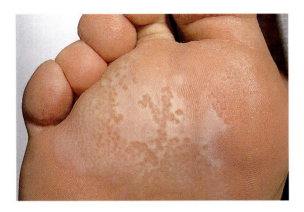

Figure 3.49

Pitted keratolysis.

Erysipelas

This is an acute streptococcal infection that typically begins as an acute systemic severe flu-like illness as the bacterium enters a fissure or other skin damage on the body — on the foot this is typically via a toe web space (Figure 3.50). Spread proximally of a wave of erythema may ascend to midcalf within 12–16 hours. One attack usually clears spontaneously within 3–4 days. Recurrent attacks may cause chronic limb lymphatic oedema and all the skin consequences of this. Prophylactic penicillin V 500 mg twice daily prevents recurrences.

on weight-bearing. Severely affected areas are most commonly present in the skin over the heel and the distal transverse arch. Treatment is of the hyperhidrosis, which is often associated: topical fusidate (Fucidin cream) twice daily for 14 days or oral erythromycin 250 mg four times daily for 14 days in severe cases may be curative though relapse is common.

Erythrasma

Coral red fluorescence is seen with Wood's UV light at sites of colonization — typically the third or fourth web space. Similar colonization may occur concurrently in the inguinal area or other flexures and body folds. It is usually asymptomatic. Various bacteria and dermatophyte fungi may be found at the same time. Treatment is to keep the area dry, plus Whitfield's ointment (3 per cent salicyclic acid and 6 per cent benzoic acid), topical fusidate, or oral oxytetracycline 250 mg four times daily for 14 days.

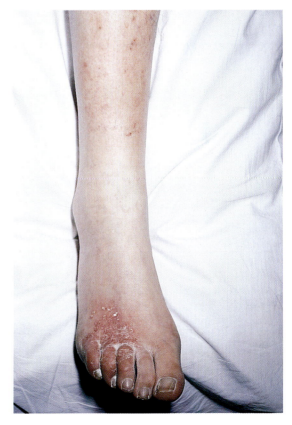

Figure 3.50

Limb showing acute erysipelas.

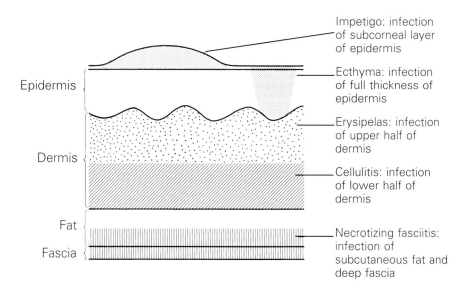

Figure 3.51

Sites and specific levels of streptococcal infections in the skin and underlying tissues.

Beta haemolytic streptococci may cause very acute, recurrent or chronic infection at different levels (Figure 3.51).

Viral infections

On the foot, the variety of lesions due to the wart virus, human papilloma virus (HPV), predominate (Figures 3.52–3.58). Though usually no more than an inconvenience, HPV infection may lead to squamous carcinoma, particularly in old and immunosuppressed individuals.

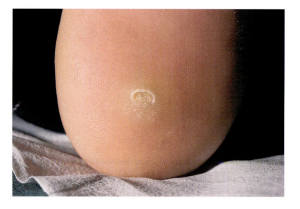

Figure 3.52

Single plantar wart (verruca).

Plantar wart (verruca)

HPV infection commonly occurs on the weight-bearing or pressure parts of the sole or toes;

the forefoot is more usually affected than the heel. There may be individual, grouped or mosaic lesions, particularly occurring in older children and young adults — direct infection during barefoot activities. Individual lesions may be asymptomatic and last only a few

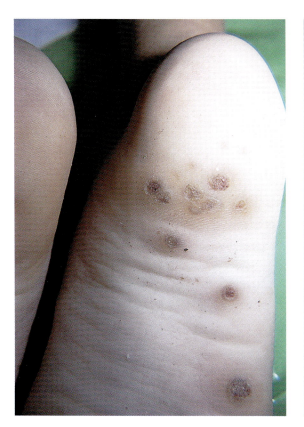

Figure 3.53
Multiple planar warts: black dots, usually associated with incipient spontaneous resolution.

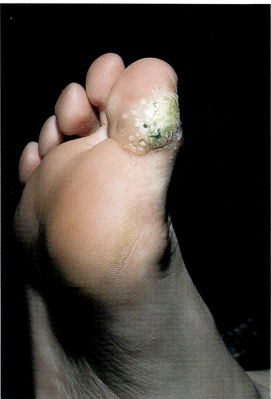

Figure 3.55
Great toe grouped warts.

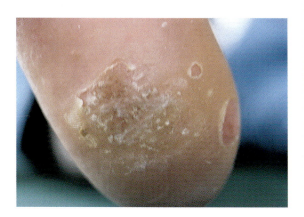

Figure 3.54
Multiple adjacent plantar (mosaic) warts.

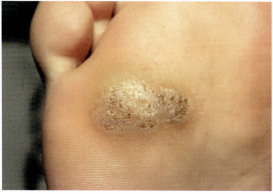

Figure 3.56
Grouped warts over metatarsal heads (usually painful at this site).

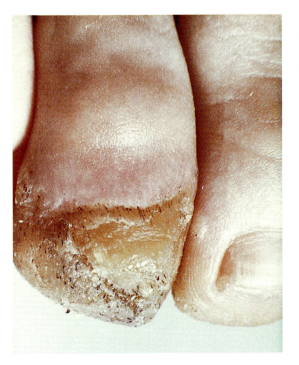

Figure 3.57
Distortion of nail apparatus by wart infection.

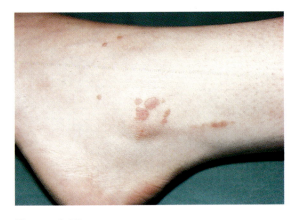

Figure 3.58
Plane warts adjacent to the lateral malleolus and the dorsum of the foot.

months. Grouped or mosaic warts may last for years and distort toe or foot function. If persistent enlarging warts last for many years, particularly in middle or old age, one must beware possible transformation into HPV-induced squamous carcinoma.

Periungual warts

These may grow and distort any part of the nail apparatus and persist for many years (Figure 3.57). Diagnosis may be difficult — similar to other tumours or swellings such as fibroma, carcinoma in situ (Bowen's disease), squamous carcinoma, or subungual corn (heloma). Note that 65 per cent remit spontaneously within two years.

Fungal infections

Tinea pedis

Tinea pedis (Latin: tinea = 'gnawing worm') is a fungal infection of the foot; toenail infection is considered in the nail disorders section (page 125). At these sites, in clinical practice, dermatophytes are the most common fungi, sometimes saprophytes ('moulds') and rarely yeasts. The genera trichophyton and epidermophyton most frequently cause foot infections, which may be severe or crippling in the immuno-compromised. It exists in three distinct patterns:

- the 'moccasin' type on the sole(s) (Figure 3.59)
- interdigital (Figure 3.60)
- vesicular spreading out from web spaces, sometimes affecting large areas of the sole and dorsum of the foot — inflamed and may mimic psoriasis or eczema (Figure 3.61).

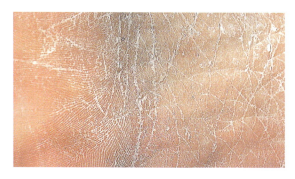

Figure 3.59

Dry 'moccasin' type of tinea pedis on the sole.

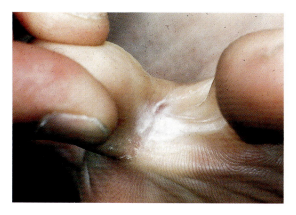

Figure 3.60

Interdigital tinea pedis.

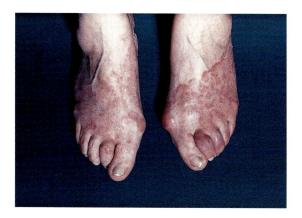

Figure 3.61

Tinea pedis: inflamed spreading variety.

Tinea pedis typically starts in the third or fourth web space, with itching, scaling and fissuring. Infection of the sole or dorsum of the foot is rare if the web spaces are normal — under these circumstances, think of other possible causes such as psoriasis or dermatitis (synonym: eczema). Trichophyton rubrum infection often gives an asymptomatic, dry 'powdery' eruption on the sole (Figure 3.59) — this may be ignored by the patient perhaps commonly presenting with onychomycosis — remember it is easier to see clear fungal microscopic changes and obtain positive culture than from nail or nail bed tissue. Chronic web space infection may be concurrently infected by pseudomonas (Figure 3.62) or candida species. Trichophyton rubrum may result in a chronic, asymptomatic, dry and powdery, red appearance of the skin of the foot. Toenail fungal infection, onychomycosis, most typically affects the big toenail alone or before other nails (see page 125).

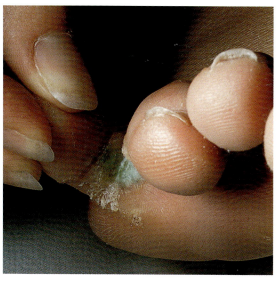

Figure 3.62

Green pseudomonas pyocyanea 'colonization' of web space.

DISORDERS OF PIGMENTATION

Disorders of pigmentation are classified as either:

- Changes in pigmentation due to melanin
- Changes in pigmentation not due to melanin.

Pigmentary changes can produce increased colour (hyperpigmentation) or decreased colour (hypopigmentation). Examples of disorders which cause changes in melanin pigmentation are given in Table 3.9.

Certain topical and systemic drugs also give rise to abnormal skin colour, for example: silver — grey-blue; gold — grey-blue; clofazamine — red; mepacrine — yellow; phenothiazines — slate grey; bismuth — grey; silver nitrate — black; potassium permanganate — brown; pyrogallic acid — brown; gentian violet — violet; dithranol — purple/brown; tar-brown; iodine — yellow/brown; eosin — red.

Pigmentary changes affecting the lower limb and foot are not unusual and are often important signs of underlying systemic disease.

Factors causing excess of melanin (hypermelanosis)

Freckles (ephelides)

Freckles are extremely common, especially in red-haired, blond and fair skinned 'celtic' people. Freckles are light brown macules usually smaller than 5 mm in diameter. They occur over a wide surface area of the body, but are more prominent on sun exposed areas where they darken on exposure to the sun, particularly on the face, shoulders and arms. The dorsum of the foot and the anterior surfaces of the legs may also be affected.

Melanocytic naevi (moles)

These are benign proliferations of melanocytes in the epidermis and dermo-epidermal junction (junctional type); sometimes also in the dermis (compound type). Most people have many melanocytic naevi distributed over their skin surface. It has been estimated that the

Table 3.9 Causes of pigmentation change.

Hypopigmentation	Hyperpigmentation
Vitiligo	Malignant melanoma
Piebaldism	Melanocytic naevus
Post-inflammatory hypopigmentation	Café au lait spots
Pityriasis versicolor	Freckles
Albinism	Malabsorption
Phenylketonuria	Renal failure Post-inflammatory hyperpigmentation Addison's disease Venous stasis Pregnancy

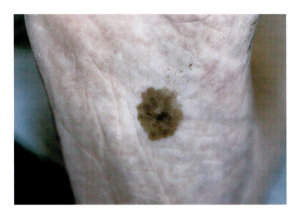

Figure 3.63
Benign pigmented (melanocytic) naevus of the sole.

average white Caucasian individual by 30 years of age has 100–150 benign naevi! The cause of these lesions is not known, although a genetic factor is likely. Most lesions appear at birth or during childhood with a sharp increase during adolescence. Lesion numbers increase less often during adulthood, although increases in numbers are sometimes seen during pregnancy. Melanocytic naevi on the foot are of the junctional type, sometimes seen on the sole of the foot or toes as circular or irregular macules. Even benign naevi on the sole or toes often have irregular outline and pigment density. If any significant change has occurred then excision is mandatory.

Café au lait spots

These are light brown oval macules which may be present at birth or develop within the first year of life. They may be associated with Von Recklinghausen's neurofibromatosis and are often seen with diffuse freckling of the armpits. Affected areas of skin appear as if coffee staining has occurred, hence the term used to describe the lesions. Von Recklinghausen's

disease is a genetic disorder characterized by the café au lait patches, axillary freckling and skin neurofibromata.

Endocrine hyperpigmentation

A number of endocrine diseases are responsible for increases in skin pigmentation; these are primarily associated with increases in production of melanocyte stimulating hormone (MSH) produced by the anterior pituitary gland. Increases in MSH production are associated with Addison's disease where the adrenal cortex becomes resistant to the action of ACTH; this causes the anterior pituitary to compensate by increasing its activity resulting in increased ACTH and MSH secretion. This pigmentation may present as multiple longitudinal pigmented streaks.

Cushing's syndrome can also cause similar changes in skin pigmentation, especially where it involves hyper-secretion of ACTH.

MSH is normally degraded by the kidney. Any long term disease of the kidney (e.g. chronic renal failure) can affect the degradation of MSH and result in hyperpigmentation.

Post-inflammatory hyperpigmentation

This condition is sometimes seen temporarily following cryosurgery and inflammatory diseases such as lichen planus. The response is thought to be related to inflammatory proteolytic enzymes activating tyrosinases in affected skin. Pigmentation is confined to a pre-existing site of inflammation, and is generally seen where inflammation has been prolonged or intense (e.g. Figure 3.35). These hyperpigmented areas typically subside and resolve over several months.

Hyperpigmentation not due to changes in melanin

Jaundice

Hepatic or biliary disease results in systemic increases in bile pigments and associated staining of the skin. The skin in jaundice appears a characteristic yellow colour. The jaundice should be taken as a sign of underlying systemic disease and investigated. The whites of the eyes and the soles of the feet may show this colour change quite early in the disease process.

Carotenaemia

Carotenaemia is due to excess carotene causing the skin to stain yellow/orange. It usually occurs secondary to renal failure as a result of failed carotene excretion. It can sometimes be seen as a result of excess dietary carotene.

Haemosiderin — deposition

Haemosiderin is due to the deposition of haemosiderin in the skin. It usually results from extravasation of erythrocytes. Erythrocytes in tissues are phagocytosed causing the release of pigment including haemosiderin and bilirubin (Figure 3.35). These pigments oxidize and stain tissues brown/red (similar to rust). Haemosiderosis most commonly affects the lower limbs, especially around the lower third of the leg and ankle, sometimes extending to the dorsum of the foot. In these cases extravasation of erythrocytes is associated with chronic venous stasis and venous hypertension. Haemosiderosis itself is clinically insignificant, but is a useful indicator of underlying pathology, and helps to identify patients at risk of stasis eczema or ulceration. Generalized 'haemosiderosis' may be a surface sign of liver or other serious internal disease.

Hypopigmentation

Disorders which cause a decrease of skin pigment and lightening of the skin are either due to absent or damage melanocytes, or alterations of tyrosine metabolism. Lack of melanocytes/melanin in the skin leaves the skin susceptible to damage from UV radiation. Premature ageing, severe sun burns, and increased risk of skin cancer are associated with hypopigmentation of 'regularly exposed areas'.

Chemical damage

Certain chemicals, including substituted phenols, destroy melanocytes. Workers in the rubber industry are exposed to such chemicals, and inadequate skin protection, including footwear, can result in patches of hypopigmentation.

Piebaldism

Piebaldism is an autosomal dominant inherited disorder, characterized by a white forelock of hair and patches of hypopigmented skin on the limbs, trunk and face. Affected individuals present with these characteristic features from birth.

Vitiligo

The term 'vitiligo' has its origins in the latin vitellus meaning 'veal-like' or 'light flesh'. It is a polygenic inherited syndrome with an incidence of 0.5–1 per cent (Figure 3.64). It most commonly begins in late childhood or early adult life. There are two main types of vitiligo; common generalized vitiligo and segmental vitiligo. The common generalized type is characterized by sharply demarcated irregular white patches. Affected areas include backs of the hands, wrists, scalp and beard and the knees. Occasionally the dorsum of the foot may be affected. Generalized vitiligo is thought to involve an auto-immune response, and is common in patients with other concurrent auto-immune disease (e.g. rheumatoid arthritis, hypothyroidism, pernicious anaemia, diabetes mellitus). It may only affect one anatomical site but typically spreads symmetrically over several years.

Segmental vitiligo is less common, and produces similar patches of white skin but segmentally distributed rather than generalized. Spontaneous remission is more likely with segmental vitiligo than with the generalized type. Potent topical steroids (e.g. dermovate, Glaxo) and narrow-band UVB may give temporary or permanent remission if used in the early stages of the disease.

Pityriasis versicolor

This disorder is characterized by ill-defined areas of hypopigmentation typically on the upper trunk. Affected skin is often scaly and dry, and may be slightly pruritic. The disorder is caused by the yeast pityrosporum orbiculare and not due to dermatophyte fungi. The carboxylic acids released by the years inhibit melanin synthesis after exposure to sunlight. Distribution is therefore confined to the upper trunk where it is a commensal organism but may also affect the limbs and dorsum of the feet, particularly in AIDS and other causes of immunosuppression. Treatment with topical imidazoles or systemic itraconazole is generally curative. After eradication of the causative organism, however, depigmented areas only slowly regain their normal colour.

Hypopituitarism

Decreased synthesis or release of anterior pituitary hormones can include decreased synthesis of melanocyte stimulating hormone. This results in a progressive, generalized loss of skin colour resulting from decreased melanin production.

Albinism

Albinism is a relatively rare disorder with an incidence of 1 : 20,000. It is an autosomal recessive trait causing abnormal synthesis of melanin. Affected individuals have normal numbers of melanocytes, but have defects in

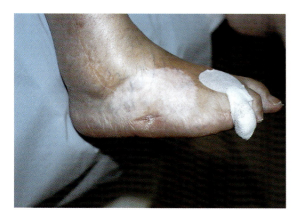

Figure 3.64
Vitiligo: sharply marginated white area.

melanin synthesis due to mutation of the gene coding for tyrosine. Albino skin is uniformly white across the whole skin surface, with pigment also lacking in hair and eyes. Freckles may be present widely distributed across the skin. Poor sight and photophobia are consequences of pigment lack in the eyes. Albinos have an increased risk of sunburn, skin cancers and cataracts. Use of high protection sun screens and UV-filtered spectacles are necessary to reduce these risks.

Phenylketonuria

This is a rare (1 : 25,000) autosomal recessive disorder which results in deficiency of the liver enzyme phenylalanine hydroxylase which catalyses the conversion of phenylalanine to tyrosine. Patients with phenylketonuria therefore have difficulty forming melanin, and have correspondingly light skin and hair. Like albinos, phenylketonurics are susceptible to skin cancer and sunburn. Individuals affected may also develop eczema and photosensitivity. High phenylalanine levels may also cause damage to the brain with extrapyramidal manifestations including athetosis and retardation.

Post-inflammatory hypopigmentation

In contrast to post-inflammatory hyperpigmentation, the loss of pigment in skin is more likely following chronic or more severe inflammation (Figure 3.65). Cryosurgery of the foot is a particular cause of depigmentation, especially if excessive tissue damage has occurred. The problem is most significant in dark skinned individuals and dark skinned races including those of black African or Asian origin. Other causes of severe inflammation affecting the

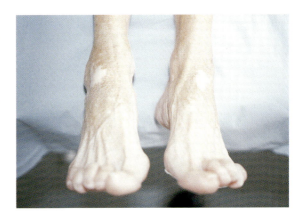

Figure 3.65
Post-eczematous hypopigmentation: anterior surface of ankles.

foot may include chronic eczema, psoriasis, sarcoidosis and lupus erythematosus.

Patches of post-inflammatory hypopigmentation are extremely common on the shins associated with 'stasis' eczema in patients with venous hypertension.

BLISTERING DISORDERS

A variety of conditions may present with vesicles, pustules or bullae of the feet. These may have a local cause or effects; or if potentially generalized, they may pose special problems to foot function. Vesicles are fluid filled sacs of less than 5 mm diameter, bullae are fluid filled sacs of greater than 5 mm diameter and pustules are lesions containing purulent material. The term blister is often used to refer to all these fluid filled lesions. It is important to note that diseases causing vesicles or bullae may become purulent, with secondary bacterial infection; also — not all pustular diseases are infective, e.g. pustular psoriasis. In clinical terms, blistering diseases may present with only erosions if the roof of individual blisters has been lost. Blisters occurring on the foot may arise as a result of confined localized pathology or as a result of more widespread systemic disease. Examples of conditions leading to formation of blisters on the foot are given in Table 3.10.

Causes of blisters arising on the feet and examples are given in Table 3.11. (Epidermolysis bullosa is added in several places because of different subtypes with varying significance).

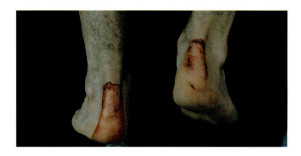

Figure 3.66

'Friction and shear' mechanical blisters in a marathon runner.

Table 3.10 Localized and generalized types of blistering eruptions occurring on the foot.

Blisters due to localized, confined cause	Blisters due to widespread, systemic cause
Burns and scalds	Epidermolysis bullosa
Cold (cryosurgery)	Diabetes mellitus
Friction blisters	Dermatitis herpetiformis (rarely feet)
Pompholyx — eczema of hands and feet	Chickenpox
Localized allergic response	Erythema multiforme
Tinea pedis	Drug eruptions
	Pemphigoid (rarely feet)
	Pemphigus (rarely feet)

Table 3.11 Causes of blistering on the feet.

Cause	Examples
Trauma	Heat — burns, scalds
(Figure 3.66)	Cold — cryosurgery
	Mechanical — pressure shear and friction blisters
	Epidermolysis bullosa
	Chemical — acid/alkali burns, drug eruptions
Infection	Herpes simplex
	Tinea pedis
	Impetigo
Immunological	Insect bite 'allergy'
	Epidermolysis bullosa
	Pompholyx
	Pemphigus
	Pemphigoid
Idiopathic	Psoriasis
	Erythema multiforme
Genetic	Epidermolysis bullosa

The diagnosis of blistering on the foot is dependent upon a thorough general approach to assessment of the patient. This assessment should include evaluation of the following:

- concurrent illnesses
- drug therapy
- family history
- previous blistering episodes
- distribution
- size
- occupation, hobbies, activities
- footwear appraisal

- orthopaedic/biomechanical evaluation
- course and development of lesion(s)
- onset and duration of lesion(s).

Blisters are classified according to their level in relation to the epidermis (Figure 3.67): superficial — occurring in stratum granulosum/corneum, thin 'roof' easily ruptured; intra-epidermal — occurring in deeper epidermal layers, thin roof, easily ruptured; sub-epidermal — occurring at dermo-epidermal junction, tense, thick roof, less easily ruptured (Figure 3.68).

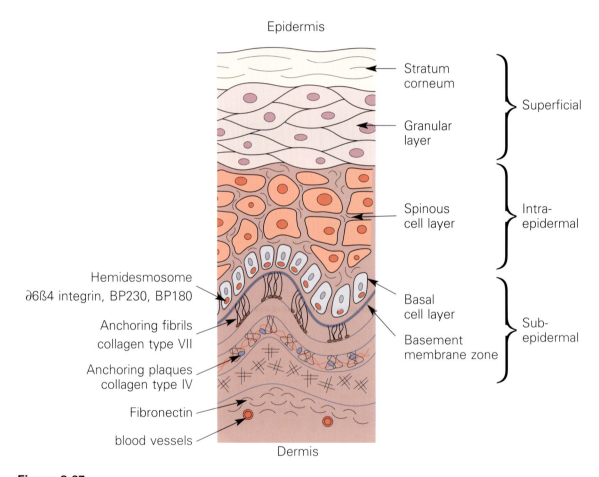

Figure 3.67

The various sites of breakdown and blister formation in congenital and acquired blistering eruptions.

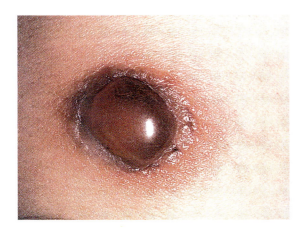

Figure 3.68
Sub-epidermal (intact) blister sometimes produced by cryosurgery.

Various histopathological changes occur with blistering including: acantholysis — loss of inter-cellular and adhesion in the prickle cell layer; spongiosus — accumulation of inter- and intra-cellular fluid and oedema; epidermolysis — damage to dermo-epidermal junction (with sub-epidermal blisters) especially; epidermal cell necrosis vacuolation and swelling of damaged cells, cellular destruction.

Localized blistering conditions of the foot

Friction blisters

Usually superficial or intra-epidermal, these blisters arise as a result of mechanical forces acting on the foot exceeding the tolerance of the inter-cellular junctions. The term 'friction blister' is really a misnomer since friction alone is rarely sufficient to cause blistering. Most friction blisters are the result of a combination of excessive friction and shear forces acting on the skin (Figure 3.66). They are more likely to arise where the resilience and resistance of skin to mechanical forces are reduced. For example:

- hyperhidrosis
- ageing
- ischaemia (see page 48)
- topical or oral steroid treatment.

The mechanical/orthopaedic deformities which predispose to formation of corns and calluses also predispose to friction blister formation (see page 33).

Severe sub-epidermal friction blisters arise where the shear forces acting on the skin of the foot are intense or prolonged. These blisters are more tense, painful and are often filled with blood. These severe blisters are also more likely to heal by scarring. They are sometimes seen in athletes including long distance runners (Figure 3.66), particularly where footwear is inadequate.

Pompholyx

The term pompholyx means a 'bubble' which is a good description for these lesions which appear acutely as clear blisters on the fingers, palms and/or the soles of the feet and toes (see page 76). Blistered areas are usually itchy, extensive and persistent. The cause is unknown but atopic individuals are prone to this condition. It may be exacerbated by heat, emotional upset of type IV allergic response. Pompholyx occasionally complicates tinea pedis infection.

Tinea pedis

Skin infection with dermatophyte fungi such as trichophyton mentagrophytes, trichophyton interdigitale or epidermophyton floccosum commonly result in recurrent episodes of inflammation with vesico-pustules of the affected areas of the foot (see page 71). Usually the sole of the foot is affected. Vesicles are extremely superficial and rupture easily. For this reason vesicles are usually only apparent on non-weight-bearing areas such as the medial longitudinal arch where the ground reaction forces have not ruptured them. In contrast to pustular psoriasis the vesico-pustules are typically at the margin of the affected areas. Recurrent vesiculation and rupture leads to accumulation of moisture in the skin which can predispose to secondary bacterial infection. This is a particular problem for those with diminished resistance to infection, including patients with diabetes mellitus, HIV infection, and patients on systemic steroid and immunosuppressive therapy.

Localized allergic response (Figure 3.69)

Exposure of the skin to surface allergens can result in type IV hypersensitivity reactions which ultimately produce blistering in associa-tion with allergic contact dermatitis (page 99). Common allergens affecting the foot include chromates used in leather tanning, leather dyes, adhesives such as epoxy resins, topical medicaments, and metals used in shoe construction. Blisters which result occur over a well demarcated area corresponding to exposure to the allergen. Extensive inflamma-tion and itching is usually prevalent. Blisters are normally small and superficial and rupture easily. Rupture leads to an exudative appear-ance and can predispose to secondary bacter-ial infection. Persistent contact with a locally applied allergen may lead to widespread dermatitis.

Burns and scalds

Thermal damage to skin can lead to large areas of damage and necrosis. Blisters occur as a result of direct thermal damage to the epider-mis. Blisters may be either superficial, intra-epidermal or sub-epidermal dependent on the extent of thermal damage. Severe burns result in exudation and fluid loss. Scarring is likely with sub-epidermal blisters following severe thermal trauma to skin.

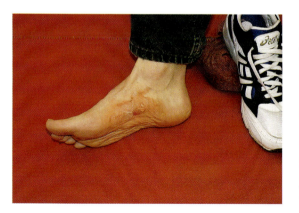

Figure 3.69
Blistering due to allergy to adhesive in sole.

Widespread/systemic causes of blistering affecting the foot

Bullous pemphigoid

Pemphigoid is an auto-immune disease with IgG antibodies binding at the dermo-epidermal junction (Figures 3.70–3.72). Complement components (mainly C3) cause inflammatory cells to be drawn to the area. Bullous pemphigoid predominantly affects the elderly. Widespread chronic blisters form typically associated with erythematous/urticated patches. There is sometimes a prodromal phase mimicking pompholyx or other types of pruritic eruption. The foot is sometimes affected. The disease is sometimes complicated by dehydration occurring with widespread fluid loss from ruptured bullae. However, the disease usually spontaneously resolves within a few years. During acute phases patients may require oral prednisolone with or without immunosuppressive agents. Long term low dose prednisolone is often required to prevent relapse of acute episodes.

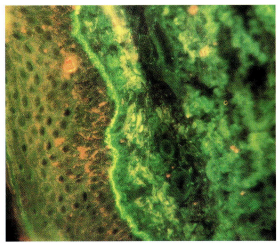

Figure 3.72
Direct immunofluorescence showing pemphigoid autoantibody linear band (bright green) at the dermoepidermal junction.

Focal or less active phases may be adequately controlled by topical steroid therapy such as dermovate ointment twice daily; or oral nicotinamide. Many cases undergo spontaneous remission within 4–5 years.

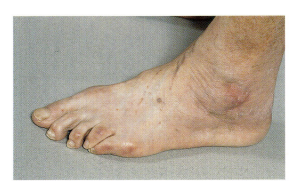

Figure 3.70
Small blisters due to bullous pemphigoid.

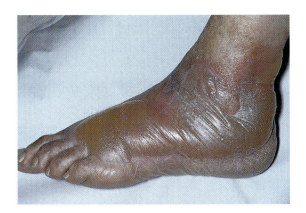

Figure 3.71
Large bullae due to bullous pemphigoid.

Pemphigus

Pemphigus is a potentially life threatening skin disorder: blisters within arise as a result of an auto-immune (IgG antibody-mediated) response to intercellular areas within the epidermis. The binding of IgG causes the keratinocytes to produce a proteolytic enzyme which digests the intercellular cement (Figures 3.73a, b). Keratinocytes lose their attachments with surrounding cells, acantholysis forms with resultant blister formation. The majority of patients develop mucous membrane lesions at some stage. Application of shearing stress to normal skin or pressure on an existing blister

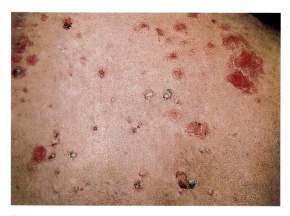

(a)

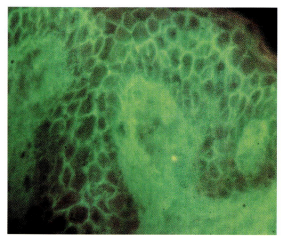

(b)

Figure 3.73

(a) Pemphigus: typically shows erosions because the blister is superficial and intraepidermal.
(b) Pemphigus: immunofluorescence showing pale green intercellular autoantibody.

causes new blister formation (Nikolsky's sign).

Blisters erode to produce exudative, painful lesions. Erosions are often complicated by infection. Patients require long term treatment with prednisolone and immunosuppressive agents. The side effects of the necessary

steroid and immunosuppresive therapy may be deleterious long term.

Erythema multiforme

Erythema multiforme is usually an adverse reaction to a drug or infection (e.g. herpes simplex or orf). It is also sometimes seen in pregnancy or patients with a variety of internal malignancies. The palms, soles, legs and arms are often affected by erythematous circular non-scaling lesions like 'targets', each lesion showing central oedema haemorrhage or blister formation. Lesions enlarge, but clear centrally. Occasionally lesions may blister. Lesions continue to occur for 1–2 weeks, or until the causative factor has been eliminated. Once lesions have cleared, areas of hyperpigmentation may remain for a few weeks. Erythema multiforme is best treated by identification and treatment of the causative factor. In cases where this is not possible topical and/or systemic steroids may be necessary. A particularly severe form of erythema multiforme (Stevens–Johnson syndrome) can cause fever and widespread severe mucosal lesions. The feet are usually spared in these cases.

Dermatitis herpetiformis

Dermatitis herpetiformis is a very itchy vesicular disease characterised by multiple, small, subepidermal vesicles. Deposits of IgA and complement components underneath the basement membrane are responsible for inducing inflammation leading to separation of the epidermis from the dermis. The disease is associated with gluten sensitivity, although patients may lack gastro-intestinal symptoms. The vesicles occur in groups, typically arising over the elbows, knees, buttocks and shoulders. Because of the itching and scratching, intact blisters may not be evident clinically. The condition is treated with oral dapsone which works within days. A gluten-free diet is also necessary since uncontrolled gluten enteropathy may lead to intestinal lymphoma (rare). The feet are rarely affected, but the condition should be suspected where widespread small, itchy, grouped ('herpetiform') blisters are present.

Epidermolysis bullosa

Epidermolysis bullosa (EB) consists of a group of diseases characterized by an increased tendency for the skin to blister, i.e. a mechanobullous disorder (Figures 3.74–3.77). They are inherited disorders, mostly showing lesions at birth or during childhood. The most common type of epidermolysis bullosa is a simple epidermolysis bullosa which affects the feet and less commonly the hands. Ill-fitting footwear makes blisters more likely, as does

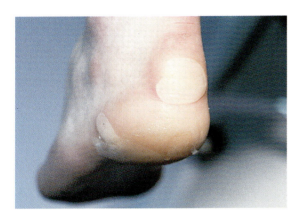

Figure 3.74
Epidermolysis bullosa: intact bulla.

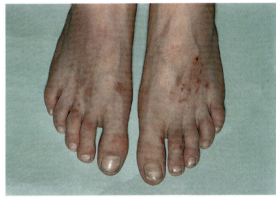

Figure 3.76
Epidermolysis bullosa: erosions.

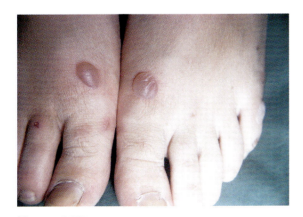

Figure 3.75
Epidermolysis bullosa: intact bulla on dorsum of feet.

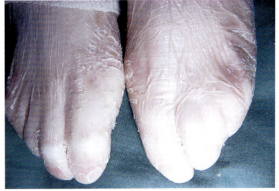

Figure 3.77
Epidermolysis bullosa: severe scarring, recessive type.

abnormal foot function and hyperhidrosis. Blisters show the same appearance as normal friction blisters or erosions, and occur at sites of increased shear or friction (Figures 3.74–76). They heal like normal friction blisters. Simple epidermolysis bullosa is the mildest form of the disease, and many patients may not seek treatment simply accepting 'inconvenience'. Modern sports science and footwear technology has greatly helped such patients to lessen the impact of the disease.

Autosomal recessive dystrophic epidermolysis bullosa is a particularly severe form of the disease. It is fortunately rare. Sub-epidermal blisters occur which fill with blood and heal with scarring. Hands and feet are commonly affected, nails become lost and webs form between the fingers and toes (Figure 3.77). Treatment is difficult and disappointing, and it is important to protect the skin of the hands and feet from trauma.

Other forms of epidermolysis bullosa tend not to affect the feet to the same extent as the two variants described above.

Epidermolysis bullosa acquisita

Epidermolysis bullosa acquisita is a variant of epidermolysis bullosa but is usually seen in middle or old age. Typically the disorder occurs in a similar pattern to simple epidermolysis bullosa, with blisters commonly occuring on the feet and hands.

Diabetic bullae

Development of intradermal tense blisters is occasionally seen in diabetes. Typically the lesion are seen on the feet and legs with a rapid onset. They are often associated with ketoacidosis but can also appear spontaneously.

BENIGN AND MALIGNANT SKIN LESIONS

In dermatology practice, the proportion of the workload often called 'lumps and bumps' has risen considerably during the last 20 years. If one includes the variety of cystic and adventitious gland lesions and benign and malignant tumours this is now over 50 per cent of the work in many parts of the world. Here we consider those that may present on the foot; or lesions that may affect many sites but have particular problems when present on the foot. Nail tumours and cysts are considered in the nail chapter.

Most skin tumours are benign, often being only a 'cosmetic nuisance'. However, it is

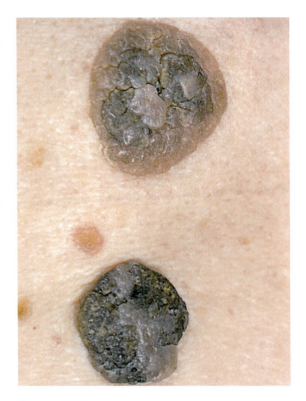

Figure 3.78
Benign seborrhoeic keratoses.

Table 3.12 Outline of tumours, naevi and swellings of skin.

A. Epidermis

Benign
- Seborrhoeic keratosis
- Keratoacanthoma
- Clear cell acanthoma
- Tumours of skin appendages, e.g. sweat glands, sebaceous glands, hair follicles
- Epidermal cysts

Dysplastic/malignant
- Basal cell carcinoma
- Actinic (solar) keratosis
- Squamous cell carcinoma: in situ (Bowen's disease), invasive
- Paget's disease
- Tumours of skin appendages

B. Melanocytes

Benign
- Freckle and lentigo

Dysplastic/malignant
- Dysplastic naevus
- Lentigo maligna
- Malignant melanoma: superficial spreading; nodular; acral

C. Dermis

Benign
- Fibrous tissue: dermatofibroma
- 'Neural' tissue, e.g. neurofibroma
- Vascular tissue: angioma/angiokeratoma; pyogenic granuloma; glomus tumour

Dysplastic/malignant
- Fibrosarcoma
- Neurofibrosarcoma
- Angiosarcoma, including Kaposi's sarcoma

D. Pseudo-tumours
- Hypertrophic and keloid scars

E. Lymphomata
- Cutaneous T-cell lymphoma (mycosis fungoides)
- Cutaneous B-cell lymphoma

F. Extension from deep tissues

G. Metastatic tumours

important to distinguish these from malignant or potentially malignant tumours quickly and effectively; decisions about what should be done about a lesion can only be made after a diagnosis has been made. The skin is a complex organ, with both benign and malignant tumours described for every component. Table 3.12 presents a simplified version of the great variety of skin tumours which may occur: the commonest are considered below.

Seborrhoeic keratosis (syn: seborrhoeic wart; basal cell papilloma) (Figure 3.78) are most frequent in the elderly, and may be solitary or multiple. Occasionally there are hundreds of lesions which may be familial. They typically consist of flat-topped areas of skin with a 'stuck-on' appearance. They may be pale, but are usually pigmented. The surface is often said to be 'greasy', but a more useful sign is small surface pits and irregularities, giving the surface a rough granular look. The differential diagnosis includes melanoma, therefore any doubt demands a biopsy; or excision if the lesion is small.

Keratoacanthoma is a self-healing, rapidly-growing tumour with histological changes of squamous carcinoma appearance. Within weeks it may grow to 3–4 cm diameter with the surface nodulation having a central keratin plug. Since there are no absolutely diagnostic signs to differentiate this tumour from squamous carcinoma, in practice most are removed.

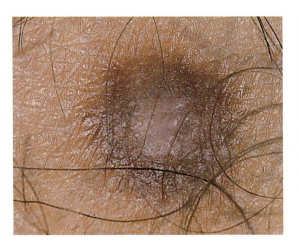

Figure 3.79
Benign dermatofibroma.

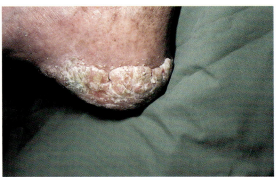

Figure 3.80
Squamous carcinoma: type known as carcinoma cuniculatum.

Epidermal cysts may be initiated from several sites in the skin:

- pilar or trichihemmal cysts from hair follicles, rare on the foot
- freckles (ephelides) – see page 72.

Dermatofriboma (Figure 3.79) are composed of fibrous tissue, (probably a reactive benign tumour), histologically more common on the lower limb in women, particularly so in pregnancy. Many erupt as a 'chronic' non-specific response to a variety of biting insects.

Angiomas both congenital and acquired types may be seen, mostly of capillary or venous origin. The congenital ones may be flat — port-wine stain type; or nodular, the 'strawberry mole' variety which may continue to enlarge for the first 3 years of life before regressing spontaneously.

Pyogenic granuloma grow at the site of minor injury as enlarging fragile bleeding lesions — like granulation tissue but histologically showing proliferating capillary — venular vessels and chronic inflammatory cells, with some fibroblastic proliferation. If the diagnosis is in doubt excision is mandatory to 'exclude' malignant tumours, e.g. squamous carcinoma, amelanotic melanoma; Kaposi's sarcoma.

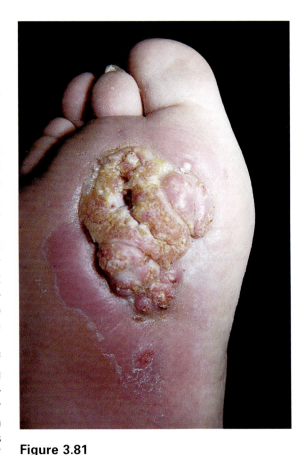

Figure 3.81
Squamous carcinoma: may be due to human papilloma virus (HPV).

Hypertrophic scars and keloids are exuberant scar tissue ('lumpy' scar) limited within the bounds of the preceding injury, operation or severe inflammation is called hypertrophic scar; mainly in Afro-Caribbean skin, similar 'causes' may lead to massive 'tumour-type' growth, e.g. ear-piercing may cause 'walnut or even small orange-sized' growth on the earlobe. Keloids may itch or be quite painful.

Basal cell carcinoma, carcinoma-in-situ and invasive squamous cell carcinoma (Figures 3.80, 3.81) are rare on the foot but must be considered in any slowly growing scaly plaque or erosion; or any irregularly growing or wart-like lesion – particularly in the middle-aged or elderly in whom common warts are relatively rare. *Carcinoma cuniculatum* is an exophytic, slowly growing 'tumour' possibly transformed from wart virus infection (Figure 3.80).

Benign solar keratoses may be seen on the exposed parts of the dorsum of the foot in white skinned individuals — only after much long-term sun exposure to the site.

'Changing' black or brown macular or palpable skin lesions need careful assessment to diagnose or disprove malignant melanoma. It is well-known that 'acral' malignant melanoma — foot, toe or nail apparatus, have a relatively poor prognosis, e.g. nail apparatus melanoma has a 5-year survival of less than 50 per cent!

Acquired melanocytic lesions are very common, particularly in white-skinned individuals. Sub-types include:

Acquired melanocytic naevi (Figure 3.82) are the familiar 'moles' and present in a number of different ways depending on the type of cells and the depth in the skin.

Junctional naevi are flat macules with melanocytes proliferating along the dermo-epidermal border.

Compound naevi have pigmented naevus cells at the dermo-epidermal border and in the dermis, producing a raised brown lesion. The dermal melanocytes may accumulate around the skin appendages and blood vessels and form a band of cells without melanin or more deeply penetrating strands of spindle cells. Proliferating naevus cells may throw the overlying epidermis into folds, giving a papillary appearance.

In a purely *intradermal naevus* the junctional element is lost, with the deeper cells showing characteristics of neural tissue. Other types of acquired pigmented naevi include:

Blue naevus is a collection of deeply pigmented melanocytes situated deep in the dermis, which accounts for the deep slate-blue colour.

Spitz naevus presents as a fleshy pink papule usually in children. It is composed of large spindle cells and epitheloid cells with occasional giant cells, arranged in 'nests'. It is benign and the old name of juvenile melanoma should be abandoned.

Halo naevus consists of a melanocytic naevus with a surrounding halo of depigmentation associated with the presence of antibodies against melanocytes in some cases. The whole naevus gradually fades in time.

Freckles or ephelides (see page 72).

Dysplastic naevus syndrome is the presenting of multiple pigmented naevi which occur, predominantly on the trunk, becoming numerous during adolescence. They vary in size —

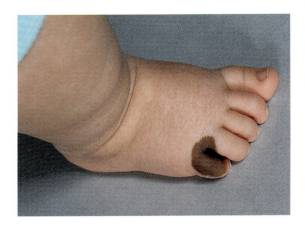

Figure 3.82
Benign pigmented naevus.

many being over 0.5 cm — and may develop malignant melanoma, particularly if there is a family history of this condition.

Congenital pigmented naevi are present at birth, generally over 1 cm in diameter, and vary from pale brown to black in colour. They often become hairy and more protuberant, possibly with an increased risk of malignant change. Larger lesions can cover a considerable area of the skin and their removal may present a considerable problem.

Malignant melanoma, these clinical types include the superficial spreading (horizontal growth phase) and nodular (vertical growth) types.

Acral melanoma occurs on the palm or sole or near or under the nails (Figures 3.83, 3.84). Benign pigmented naevi may also occur in these sites and it is important to recognize early dysplastic change in such lesions. A very important indication that discolouration of the nail is due to melanoma is Hutchinson's sign — pigmentation of the nail fold adjacent to the nail. It is important to distinguish *talon noir*, in which a black area appears on the sole or heel. It is the result of trauma — for example, sustained while playing squash — causing haemorrhage into the dermal papillae (Figure 3.85). Paring the skin gently with a scalpel will

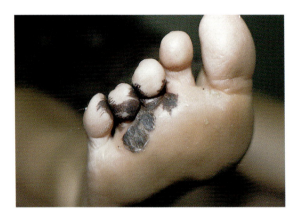

Figure 3.83
Acral melanoma: superficial spreading type.

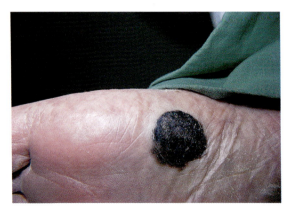

Figure 3.84
Acral melanoma: nodular variety.

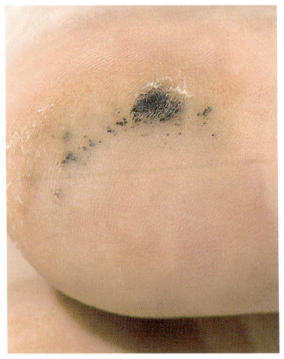

Figure 3.85
Black heel, due to acute pressure on the heel in a squash-player (capillary haemorrhage).

reveal distinct blood filled papillae, to the relief of doctor and patient alike.

Other types of melanoma. As the melanoma cells become more dysplastic and less well differentiated they lose the capacity to produce melanin and form an *amelanonitic melanoma*. Such non-pigmented nodules may easily be regarded as harmless but are in fact extremely dangerous.

To 'filter out' malignant melanoma from benign pigmented lesions the following questions are important:

- Is an existing mole getting larger or a new one growing? After puberty moles usually do not grow (this sign essentially refers to adults). Remember that naevi may grow rapidly in children
- Does the lesion have an irregular outline? Ordinary moles are a smooth regular shape
- Is the lesion irregularly pigmented? Particularly, is there a mixture of shades of brown and black?
- Is the lesion larger than 1 cm in diameter?
- Is the lesion inflamed or is there a reddish edge?
- Is the lesion bleeding, oozing or crusting?
- Does the lesion itch or hurt?

Any pigmented lesion, whether newly arising or already present, which exhibits three

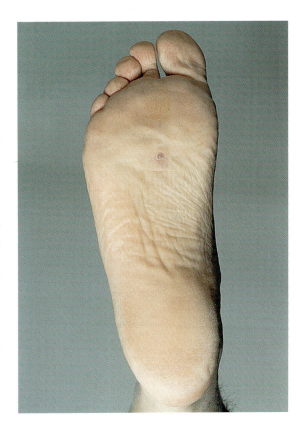

Figure 3.87
Benign eccrine poroma of the sole.

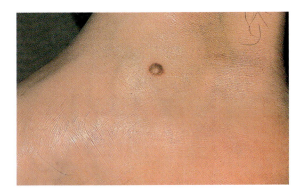

Figure 3.86
Dermatofibroma.

or more of the seven listed features, and especially one of the first three, should be treated as highly suspicious. However, most lesions will be benign, e.g. dermatofibroma (Figure 3.86).

Eccrine poroma (Figure 3.87) is a benign tumour arising from the eccrine duct epithelium in the region of the dermo-epidermal junction, usually presenting as a solitary lesion on the sole or the palm. The well-demarcated outgrowth is mainly reddish-pink in colour, sometimes with surrounding hyperpigmentation, and up to 2 cm in diameter. Differential diagnosis is from amelanotic malignant melanoma and squamous carcinoma. Treatment is by surgical excision.

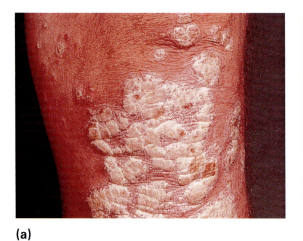

(a)

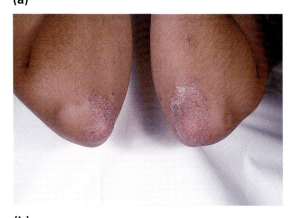

(b)

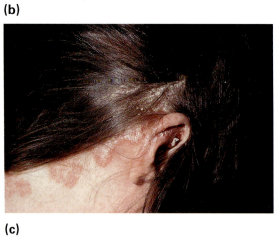

(c)

Figure 3.88

Common sites for psoriasis: **(a)** knees;
(b) elbows; **(c)** scalp.

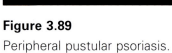

Figure 3.89

Peripheral pustular psoriasis.

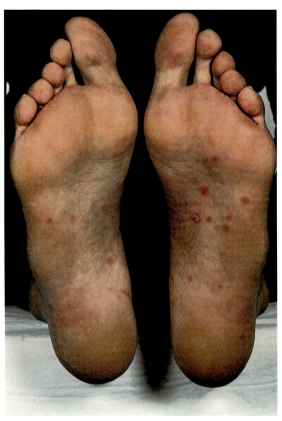

Figure 3.90

Symmetrical hyperkeratotic psoriasis of the
soles.

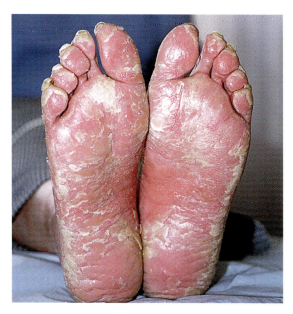

Figure 3.91
Soles of the feet in exfoliative erythrodermic psoriasis.

Kaposi's sarcoma is a malignant vascular tumour which merits special mention in spite of its rarity. 'Classical' Kaposi's sarcoma occurs in Ashkenazi Jews and northern Italians. A much more aggressive form is seen in Africans and in patients with the acquired immunodeficiency syndrome (AIDS). The clinical features consist of purplish plaques and nodules. Sites of predilection include legs in the classical form; anywhere in the aggressive form. The differential diagnosis is from other vascular lesions.

Lymphomas the lymphomatous involvement of the skin may be secondary, e.g. in non-Hodgkin's B-cell lymphoma. However, the skin may be the original site, especially in cutaneous T-cell lymphoma (often called 'mycosis fungoides'). The clinical features are variable; some areas remain unchanged or grow slowly for years; red, well-circumscribed, scaly plaques and tumours eventually develop. The differential diagnosis is from eczema or psoriasis.

One can conclude that if there is any clinical doubt with regard to the lesions described in this chapter then histological confirmation is mandatory.

PSORIASIS

Psoriasis may classically have widespread skin signs, it sometimes presents as a foot problem (Figures 3.88–3.91). It is imperative that podiatrists should recognize the signs at other sites since the foot signs will not always be diagnostic when viewed alone. It is a very common disorder, and has been estimated to affect 2 per cent of the population. The exact cause of psoriasis is unknown but it is thought that genetic factors play an important role. However, other factors are necessary in the clinical expression of the disease. Only one third of patients with psoriasis have a family history of the complaint in a first degree relative. It would appear that the predisposition for the disease is inherited and other factors 'precipitate' the disorder. The known triggers for psoriasis include streptococcal infections, trauma to the skin, severe mental stress, and certain drugs, e.g. oral lithium salts used in psychiatry and chloroquine. However, these trigger factors are only found in a minority of patients. Psoriasis is characterized by proliferation of the epidermal cells and a maturation defect of these cells, resulting in an abnormal keratin layer. There is evidence that this proliferation of cells is mediated by immunological mechanisms, probably mediated via T-lymphocytes.

Clinical features

Psoriasis affects the sexes equally. It may appear for the first time at any age, but is very rare before the age of 5, and uncommon before 15 years of age. The disorder most frequently presents in young adult life; the incidence of first presentation falls from middle age. However, the disorder may appear for the first time even in the eighth and ninth decades of life. The clinical features of psoriasis vary depending on the site of involvement, e.g. palms and soles, and flexural regions may have a different appearance to the lesions at other sites. The commoner sites of involvement are the extensor surfaces of the knees and elbows (Figures 3.88a, b), followed by the scalp (Figure 3.88c) and sacral region; but any part of the skin may be affected. The typical lesion is a well-demarcated red, raised patch with silvery white scales; the scales are loosely bound and gentle scratching shows flaking of the lesion and increases the white appearance. If all the scales are removed capillary bleeding points are seen. The extent of involvement in psoriasis varies considerably, from a few local-ized patches to total involvement of the body surface.

Scalp

Psoriasis may affect the scalp with or without lesions elsewhere (Figure 3.88c). The involve-ment varies from a solitary patch to the whole of the scalp: The lesions usually stop at the hairline. Examination shows well-demarcated patches with an irregularly thickened surface, the excess and abnormal keratin adhering to the hair.

Palms and soles

At these sites psoriases may present with discrete patches or be confluent (Figures 3.89–3.91). When the lesions are patchy they present as firm hyperkeratotic yellowish brown areas with adherent scale. If the involvement is diffuse, the palms and soles are red with overt scaling (Figure 3.91), and a sharp line of demarcation between the involved and non-involved skin at the sides of the palms and soles. Occasionally psoriasis only affects the palms and soles with no lesions elsewhere and the diagnosis can be difficult. This type may be hyperkeratotic and mainly on the weight-bearing sites (Figure 3.90).

Nails

The nails are affected in approximately 50 per cent of patients with psoriasis (page 91). The commonest feature is small uniform pits. Other features include onycholysis (distal separation of the nail plate from the nail bed), subungual hyperkeratosis and dystrophy (breaking of nail). Occasionally involvement of the nails occurs without skin lesions; in those who are athletically active, considerable subun-gual hyperkeratosis may occur.

Flexural psoriasis

When psoriasis affects the body 'folds' — groins, perianal skin and axillae, it appears as well-demarcated red areas with a shiny surface. The white dry scales are not present because of the moisture of these areas. Occasionally painful fissures may occur, partic-ularly in the posterior natal cleft.

Guttate psoriasis

This is a term used to describe the sudden appearance of numerous small lesions of psoriasis, usually predominating on the trunk. Subsequently similar lesions may appear on the limbs. The lesions are red but often have only minimal scaling. The distinctive feature of guttate psoriasis is that in the majority of patients the disorder is self-limiting, the lesions disappearing within 3 months of onset. It is most common in children and young adults. One of the known triggers is streptococcal infection.

Erythrodermic psoriasis

This is the term used when psoriasis involves the whole of the skin surface. The patient presents with erythema and scaling. However the scaling is different to that seen in plaques of psoriasis, and is not as thick and does not always have a white appearance (Figure 3.91). This may be due to the fact that erythrodermic psoriasis is the most active form of the disease, and less keratin is produced than in chronic plaque psoriasis.

Pustular psoriasis (peripheral pustulosis)

There are two types of pustular psoriasis: one is the localized form seen on the palms and soles, where the condition presents as red, scaly patches with small pustules (Figure 3.89). These lesions are sterile. Localized pustular psoriasis is usually but not always symmetrical. The condition tends to be persistent and has been termed 'persistent eruption of the palms and soles'. Whether these lesions are indeed themselves psoriatic or simply associated with the psoriatic trait is not known.

The other form of pustular psoriasis is the generalized type. In this condition sheets of small pustules appear in extensive psoriatic lesions on the trunk and limbs. The patients usually have a fever and constitutional upset. This form of psoriasis is rare.

Koebner phenomenon

This is the term applied to psoriasis appearing at the sites of trauma. It is seen after falls, cuts, thermal burns and severe sunburn. This sign is also seen in other non-infective conditions such as lichen planus and vitiligo.

Arthropathic psoriasis

Five per cent of patients with psoriasis develop arthropathy. It is similar in its distribution to rheumatoid arthritis except that the terminal interphalangeal joint is most particularly involved in psoriasis. The disorder can also be distinguished from rheumatoid arthritis by the fact that the rheumatoid factor is absent.

As in rheumatoid arthritis psoriatic involvement of the joints may be mild and self-limiting, or there may be severe involvement leading to permanent damage and deformity of the joints. The condition may also affect one or only a few joints, or there may be extensive involvement. Psoriatic arthropathy may occur without skin lesions; but only very rarely does it occur without concurrent nail signs.

Prognosis

The course of psoriasis is variable. In some the disease is limited to a few persistent patches on the elbows or knees, whilst in others the disease becomes extensive. It has been estimated that 40 per cent of patients can expect spontaneous remissions. The factors which control the extent and persistence of the lesions are not known.

Psoriasis involving only the palms and/or soles has to be distinguished from chronic eczema. The line of demarcation between the affected and non-affected skin is more marked in psoriasis. If the lesions are not confluent but present as small plaques, the condition has to be distinguished from lichen planus at these sites. The fissured inflamed plantar hyperkeratotic type is difficult to diagnose from eczema.

Nail involvement in psoriasis has to be distinguished from onychomycosis. Pits are not seen in fungal infections, but onycholysis, subungual hyperkeratosis and dystrophy may occur in both conditions. Specimens must be taken for mycology if there is doubt as to the diagnosis.

Flexural or intertriginous psoriasis may be confused with intertriginous eczema, fungal infections and erythrasma. If only the intertriginous areas are involved it may be impossible to distinguish between eczema and psoriasis. Ringworm fungal infections tend to have a raised scaly edge.

Pustular psoriasis on the palms and soles has to be distinguished from secondary infected eczema or fungal infections. If there is doubt, specimens should be taken for mycology and bacteriology. Generalized pustular psoriasis has to be differentiated from widespread impetigo, pemphigus, and a rare condition called subcorneal pustular dermatosis.

Erythroderma due to eczema has the same appearance as that due to psoriasis, and the preceding history may give the exact diagnosis. The Sezary syndrome and mycosis fungoides, which are skin reticuloses, may also give rise to erythroderma.

There is the possibility of the rash being a secondary syphilitic eruption. If there is joint involvement, serological tests for the rheumatoid factor and uric acid level should be carried out.

Table 3.13 The management of psoriasis.

Types of Psoriasis		Factors relating to the patient	Principal therapies
Type	Chronic plaque	Age	Topical treatment
	Guttate psoriasis	Work/hobbies	Tars
	Pustular psoriasis	Transport	Dithranol
Site	Scalp	Mobility	Calcipotriol
	Face		Corticosteroids
	Flexures		Retinoids
	Hands/feet		Ultraviolet radiation
	Nails		PUVA
Activity	Chronic		UVB
	Erythroderma		Systemic
	Generalized		Methotrexate
	pustular		Retinoids
			Cyclosporin
			Hydroxyurea

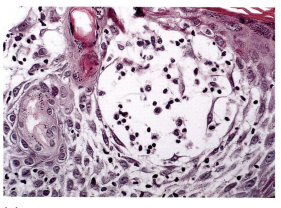

(a)

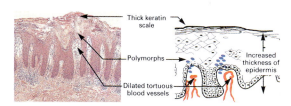

Thick keratin scale

Polymorphs

Dilated tortuous blood vessels

Increased thickness of epidermis

(b)

Figure 3.92

(a) Epidermis in acute eczema with prominent inter- and intracellular oedema and monocytic infiltrate.
(b) Epidermal 'proliferation' increased throughout the epidermis.

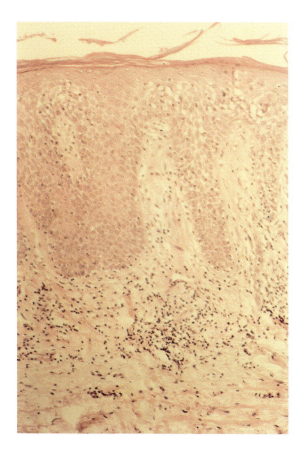

Figure 3.93

Chronic eczema (dermatitis). Diffuse oedema in the epidermis and elongation of the rete ridges, with considerable chronic inflammatory infiltrate.

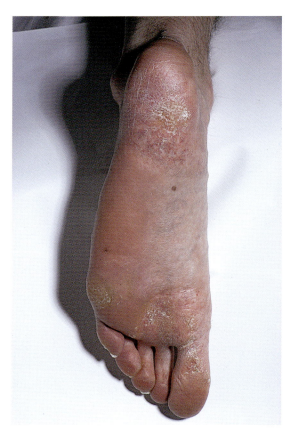

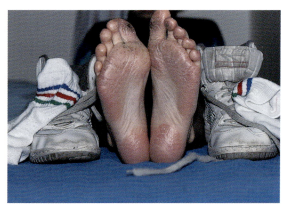

Figure 3.96
Juvenile plantar dermatosis: dry 'shiny' fissured forefoot. Atopic, but associated with 'occlusive' socks and shoes.

Figure 3.94
Vesicular 'pompholyx' eczema (atopic individual).

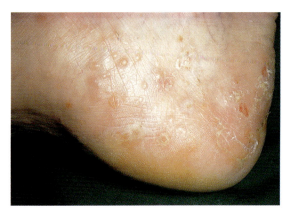

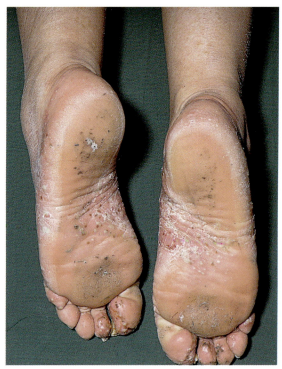

Figure 3.95
Vesicular 'pompholyx' eczema.

Figure 3.97
Plantar dermatitis with hyperkeratosis.

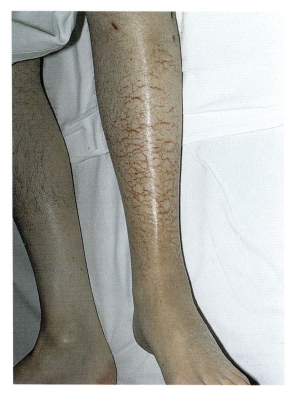

Figure 3.98
Constitutional 'asteatotic' eczema.

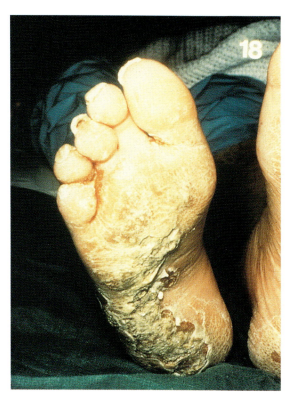

Figure 3.100
Chronic hyperkerartotic dermatitis.

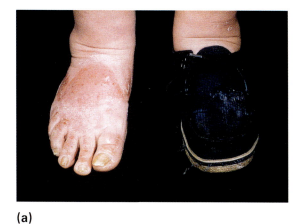

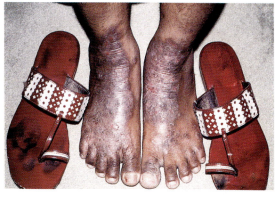

(a)

(b)

Figure 3.99
(a, b) Footwear allergy contact dermatitis.

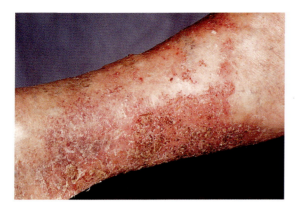

Figure 3.101

Stasis (venous) dermatitis, with secondary bacterial colonization (infection).

Management

The general management principles can be outlined as indicated in Table 3.13. It is important to explain the nature of the condition to the patient and stress the non-contagious aspect of the disorder. Patients should be told that at present no permanent cure exists, but that the condition can always be cleared and controlled if necessary, and that a large proportion will achieve a spontaneous remission.

If psoriasis is active, then whatever treatment is given the condition is likely to relapse when treatment is discontinued, whereas if the disorder is not active, a long remission may be obtained with the same treatment. The activity of psoriasis can be judged by a number of clinical features. If the condition is extensive or new lesions are developing then the disease is active, whereas if the lesions are not increasing in size and no new ones are appearing, this suggests low activity. Plaques which show clearing from the centre often imply spontaneous resolution of these lesions.

ECZEMA — DERMATITIS

'Eczema' is used synonymously with 'dermatitis'. Eczema denotes a particular inflammatory reaction in the skin which appears to have a number of different causes although the final pathogenic events are similar; the word literally means 'boiling over'.

There are essentially two groups of eczema, namely that produced by external substances, exogenous eczema, and that due to internal or constitutional factors, endogenous eczema (Figures 3.92–3.101). It is important to distinguish between these two groups; in exogenous eczema identifying the causative agent may result in a permanent cure, whilst in the case of endogenous eczema the treatment is suppressive rather than curative.

Exogenous eczema

This may be due to two groups of substances, primary irritants and allergens:

Primary irritant eczema

Irritants are chemicals which directly damage the skin, particularly the keratin which acts as a protective barrier. Once the protective function of the keratin is impaired irritant chemicals are able to pass into the cellular component of the epidermis and cause an inflammatory reaction. The chemicals causing irritant eczema are common substances both in the home and at work. In the home they include detergents, cleansers, bleaches, washing powders, soaps and solvents. At work the common ones are cutting oils, acids, alkalis and solvents. Continual wetting of the skin, e.g. in bar workers and fishmongers who do not dry the skin, may lead to evaporation of water and cooling of the skin which results in cracking of the keratin allowing penetration of irritant substances. It seems there are constitutional factors which predispose to the development of irritant eczema as certain individuals appear more prone than others. Irritant reactions are most likely on the feet with occlusive footwear and/or constant wetting.

If patients are prone to develop irritant eczema then that tendency will probably persist for life. Nevertheless, if the exposure to the irritants can be stopped or at least decreased the eventual outlook is good. It does seem, however, in certain individuals, that once eczema develops it may be some time before it is controlled despite no further contact with irritants.

Allergic contact eczema

This is caused by the skin becoming sensitized to a specific antigen, which on further exposure results in an inflammatory reaction in the skin (Figure 3.99a, b). Why some patients develop sensitivity to certain chemicals and others do not is unknown. Once patients develop sensitivity it tends to last indefinitely. There are numerous chemicals which may sensitize. A number of these substances are very common, e.g. dyes in clothing, or nickel in jewellery or any metal contact, whilst others are rare and tend to be found only in certain industrial processes.

Contact allergic eczema is rare before puberty and in the elderly, and this may be related to less vigilant cell-mediated immunity in the elderly.

The site and pattern of the eczema depends on site of contact; however, the penetration of the allergen will be more rapid through thin and moist skin. Thus when the face is exposed to an allergen the eczema will first appear around the eyes, where the skin is thinnest on

the face. Contact to the dye in tights may appear in the popliteal fossae where the skin is thinnest on the legs, or on the feet due to hydration of the keratin from sweating. The site of the eczema may well suggest the allergen; however, the nature of the allergen is not always obvious.

Contact eczema is often suggested by a sharp cut-off point between the affected and unaffected skin, the eczema only occurring at the exact sites of contact. Allergic contact eczema is often acute with intense erythema, weeping and vesiculation. However, there are variations in presentation of contact eczema, in that the eczema may spread beyond and around the site of contact. In addition allergens which are absorbed into the circulation on the sensitized lymphocytes travel to other parts of the body where eczema may appear without direct contact. This is most commonly seen with nickel, in that the eczema often appears in the antecubital fossae and around the eyes. Finally it must be remembered that any eczema may spread to other sites in a non-specific pattern, due to so-called 'autosensitization'; this occurs both with endogenous and exogenous eczema.

On the feet, endogenous eczema, psoriasis and fungal infection are the common differential diagnoses.

Allergic contact eczema is established by so-called patch tests. In this procedure the suspected substance is applied to the skin under an occlusive dressing for 48 hours. If the patient is allergic to the substance a patch of eczema will be present at the patch test site. Occasionally, however, there is a delayed reaction and the site should be inspected again after a further 48 hours. It is important to know that some substances which may act as irritants or are strong sensitisers should be diluted before being applied and occluded. If the cause of the eczema is obvious then patch tests may not be necessary.

Endogenous eczema

This specific form of skin inflammation occurs in constitutionally predisposed individuals, e.g. atopics. External factors may exacerbate the condition, but are not causative. It is best to split the endogenous eczemas into the following distinct types:

- atopic
- seborrhoeic
- discoid
- pompholyx
- lichen simplex
- asteatotic
- hypostatic/venous.

Atopic eczema

This is sometimes called 'infantile' eczema because of the usual time of onset, between ages 2 and 12 months (Figures 3.94, 3.95). About 25 per cent of the population are potentially atopic, that is, have a genetically determined predisposition to atopic eczema, asthma, rhinitis and conjunctivitis; only 5 per cent of these individuals will actually develop atopic eczema. Ninety per cent of cases clear by the age of 12, but 10 per cent recur during teenage years; most are clear by 30 years.

Although genetic factors are important in atopic eczema the pathogenetic pathways are not known, but two possible hypotheses have been put forward:

- deficiency of intestinal mucosal IgA, and
- deficiency of T-suppressor cells in early infancy.

In both cases overproduction of IgE occurs in response to excess 'untrapped' antigen.

The infantile eruption is symmetrical, affecting face and trunk, but in early childhood the eczema takes on the typical flexural distribution, including ankles and dorsum of the feet. Late onset, 'extensor' pattern, associated asthma, family and social problems are all bad prognostic indicators.

Typically lesions are red and scaly, with weeping when acute, or crusting when subacute, and thickened scaly skin when chronic. Small red papules are common and vesicles are rare. Pruritus is intense and leads to scratching. Repeated scratching causes lichenification and later excoriated papules and nodules. Post-inflammatory hypo- and hyperpigmentation are common.

The condition can be aggravated by cold and occasionally by hot, humid conditions, also by wool, cosmetics, infections and emotional stress.

Secondary infection of eczema with staphylococci or streptococci is a common problem. Children with atopic eczema are more likely to develop viral problems such as warts and molluscum contagiosum, and herpes simplex infections may disseminate to give rise to Kaposi's varicelliform eruption.

Diagnosis is usually straightforward, but some cases of seborrhoeic and contact eczema may cause confusion; distribution of the eruption and family history often provide the key.

Juvenile plantar dermatosis (dermatitis)

Sometimes called 'glazed foot' (Figure 3.96), this is more common in atopic subjects; it is characterized by a dry, fissured and scaly eruption affecting the forefoot and volar areas, occasionally extending to the heel but sparing the arch. Cases of the condition were first described some 30 years ago in parallel with the fashion of wearing plastic and synthetic materials in footwear. It normally occurs in young school children, and normally resolves by puberty. The use of cork insoles with natural fibre hosiery and emollients are of benefit.

Management

Treatment of mild cases may be easy, and 90 per cent of eczema remits in childhood; but severe cases or chronic cases can be very difficult to treat and, in addition to exacting therapy, time must be spent with the parents in order to discuss the nature of the condition and give advice, reassurance and encouragement.

Eczema is exacerbated by emotional stress, and an attack of eczema, possibly accompanied by another manifestation of atopy such as asthma, in turn creates distress thus setting up a vicious circle which is often difficult to break; counselling and helping with social problems may be more useful than drugs.

All treatment aims at keeping the skin as supple as possible. Emollients such as oilatum oils and emulsifying ointment should be added to bathing water, and soap avoided. After baths, and at other times, emollients such as E45 or aqueous cream should be applied. All these preparations act by:

- soothing
- increasing hydration of stratum corneum by reducing water lost in evaporation.

Topical steroids provide the most effective treatment. The strength, quantity and type of application depend on the severity of the eczema and the type of skin affected. The weakest dilution possible should be used in order to avoid the complications of local thinning of skin and erythema, and possible systemic effects of absorbed steroids causing adrenal suppression and stunting of growth in children.

Crude coal tar is effective in chronic eczema and may be used as a topical application but is best used mixed with emulsifying ointment (20 per cent liquor picis carb in emulsifying ointment) as a soap substitute. Coal tar impregnated bandages are useful for the legs.

It is important to treat pruritus in order to reduce distress as well as prevent excoriations and lichenifications, and oral antihistamines are used, mostly at nights, when their sedative effect is probably more important than their antipruritic effect. Trimeprazine is a popular antihistamine and more recently ketotifen has been claimed to be useful.

Seborrhoeic eczema

This is a characteristically scaly eczema affecting areas rich in sebaceous glands, or intertriginous areas, mostly scalp, alinasal folds, and flexures; only rarely is the foot affected.

Cradle cap is easily treated with a mild keratolytic such as 1 per cent sulphur and 1 per cent salicyclic acid in aqueous cream, applying in the evening two or three times per week with shampooing next morning; for mild cases simple application such as olive oil may suffice.

Infantile seborrhoeic eczema of trunk and nappy area should be treated by a mild steroid such as 1 per cent hydrocortisone, combined with nystatin in the nappy area if candida is suspected.

Emulsifying ointment should be used as a soap substitute. Nappies should be changed regularly and left off for several hours each day.

In the adult the scalp is treated in a similar way, but with stronger keratolytics; up to 5 per cent strength sulphur and salicylic acid creams and ung cocois co are commonly used. If scaling and irritation are severe, potent steroid lotion can be applied between hair washes.

Weak steroids are used for seborrhoeic eczema of the face, while trunk and intertriginous areas require moderate strength steroids. Antiseptic paints such as 1 per cent aqueous gentian violet or magenta paint can be useful in intertriginous areas as they are drying and prevent secondary infection, and topical steroids can be applied after drying of the paint.

Discoid eczema

Otherwise known as nummular eczema, this is characterized by well-defined coin-like lesions distributed symmetrically on extensor surfaces of the limbs and dorsal aspects of hands and feet. It may be associated with pompholyx eczema. The lesions are scaly plaques, and if acute may have vesicles and exude serum. They are often very itchy. The condition can occur at any age, but it is most common between the ages of 20 and 40. As well as limbs, hands and feet, nail folds can be affected causing nail ridging, and rarely the face is affected. Despite a good response to treatment, relapses tend to occur.

Management

Lesions usually respond to moderate strength steroids, but occasionally potent steroid applications are required. Antihistamines may be required for pruritus in the early stages before the eczema clears with topical steroids.

Pompholyx eczema

This is one of the most incapacitating eczemas, being localized to palms and soles and characterized by very itchy vesicles and bullae, and painful fissures (Figures 3.94, 3.95).

The condition may be associated with excess sweating, discoid eczema, nickel sensitivity and fungal infection. In nickel-sensitive subjects it has been claimed that exacerbation may be related to a recent high intake of nickel such as occurs in eating acidic fruit boiled in stainless steel saucepans (which contain small amounts of nickel).

Usually presenting in young adults, the eruption is commonly symmetrical and begins in the 'sweat' areas, i.e. palms, soles, and sides and dorsum of digits. As in other types of eczema, in severe cases eruptions may be spread to backs of hands and feet, and to the limbs.

The initial small itchy vesicles expand and coalesce to form bullae. These may dry up or persist and occasionally become secondarily infected and lead to cellulitis. In chronic pompholyx, palms and soles become dry and scaly with painful fissures, and nails become ridged if nail folds are involved. Attacks of pompholyx may be precipitated by heat or emotion, presumably mediated by excessive sweating.

Management

Acute blistering pompholyx is best treated by potassium permanganate soaks; 1:8000 for 15 minutes, three times daily. After drying, an appropriate weak steroid is applied.

Lichen simplex

This can be regarded as a localized form of atopic eczema. It occurs mainly in adults, women more commonly than men, and there is often other personal or family history of atopy.

Clinical features

The lesions are solitary, sited typically at nape of neck (less commonly on forearms, wrists, shins and ankles). Variable-size plaques are formed and itching is intense. Lichenification with exaggerated skin ridges occurs, and the lesions are often reddish purple and hyperpigmented.

Very potent topical steroids are usually required to reduce the inflammation and stop the itching. Antihistamines do not help. Intralesional steroids are effective, and occlusion with coal tar bandages is often successful.

Asteatotic eczema

This is also known as xerosis, winter itch, and eczema craquelé, and is a disease of the elderly characterized by dry cracked skin that may have been subjected to excessive bathing and scrubbing (Figure 3.98).

The skin becomes degreased by washing, and chapped (dried and cracked) by the cold. The legs, particularly the shins, are affected, and sometimes the trunk and arms.

Topical steroids diluted in white soft paraffin reduce itching and heal the skin. 'Greasing' agents such as emulsifying ointment are used as soap substitutes. Healing is usually rapid and continual use of 'greasing' agents prevents recurrence.

Hypostatic/venous eczema

This eczema occurs on the inner aspect of the shin, just above the medial malleolus, following hypostasis, i.e. poor tissue perfusion due to high venous pressure, that may result from circulatory problems, e.g. postphlebitic syndrome, or incompetent valves in the venous system of the legs (Figure 3.101).

Ulceration, secondary infection, and generally poor healing are all-too-common problems. Additionally, allergic contact and irritant eczemas can more easily develop in these areas of thin and broken skin, and may then become disseminated. Prolonged severe hypostatic eczema itself may similarly become generalized by 'autosensitization'; this is a process by which any eczema — endogenous or exogenous — can disseminate, in some patients a delayed type response to their own epidermal antigens being demonstrated. Some 'autosensitization' occurs in characteristic patterns, for example, hypostatic eczema spreading to the arms, and nickel sensitivity to the eyes; sometimes it may be difficult to differentiate between autosensitization of endogenous eczema and superimposition of allergic contact eczema.

The cause of the hypostasis must be determined and treated if possible and this may involve venography. Postural drainage to counteract the high venous pressure is helpful. At night the foot of the bed should be raised 22–23 cm (9 inches). Patients should be encouraged to lie on the bed for an hour in the afternoon. Standing and sitting with the legs down are bad for the condition, but exercise – since the muscle pump encourages venous drainage – is better. If ulceration develops this should be treated by cleaning the ulcer with equal parts eusol and paraffin, and then dressed with a non-adhesive dressing. A firm supportive bandage from the toes to the knee should be worn. Patients often find a cotton bandage impregnated with zinc oxide next to the skin under an elastoplast bandage very helpful. These bandages need only be changed weekly.

Overall treatment may be long and difficult, and a sympathetic and encouraging approach from a well co-ordinated medical team is as important as a co-operative and well motivated patient.

4 Nail disorders

INTRODUCTION
NAIL STRUCTURE AND FUNCTION AND RELATION TO FOOT FUNCTION
NAIL DYNAMICS

INTRODUCTION

Normal nails are to some degree taken for granted and their importance is only really noted when they are lost or distorted through trauma or disease — indeed abnormal nails on the feet can cause foot malfunction to a great degree. Nail structure (Figure 1.12) and function and their disorders and treatment are therefore here considered separate from the foot diseases in general.

NAIL STRUCTURE AND FUNCTION AND RELATION TO FOOT FUNCTION

The anatomy and physiology of the nail apparatus must be considered in isolation and also in relation to the rest of the foot. Many disorders of nails are either directly due to functional faults in the foot (see Chapter 2), or diseases of the nail apparatus may be modified by alterations in digital or foot shape or movement.

The nail apparatus develops from the primitive epidermis. The main function of the nail apparatus is to produce a strong, relatively inflexible nail plate over the dorsal surface of the end of each digit. The nail plate on toes acts as a protective covering for the digit. Whilst fingernails cover approximately one-fifth of the dorsal surface, on the great toe, the nail may cover up to 50 per cent of the dorsum of the digit.

Structure

The component parts of the nail apparatus are shown diagrammatically in Figure 1.12. The rectangular nail plate is the largest structure, resting on and firmly attached to the nail bed and the underlying bone, less firm proximally, apart from the postero-lateral corners. Approximately one-quarter of the nail is covered by the proximal nail fold whilst a narrow margin of the sides of the nail plate is often occluded by the lateral nail folds. Underlying the proximal part of the nail is the white lunula (syn. half-moon lunule); this area represents the most distal region of the matrix. On the foot this may only be visible on the great toes. The nail plate distal to the lunula is usually pink due to its translucency which allows the redness of the vascular nail bed to be seen through it. The proximal nail fold has two epithelial surfaces, dorsal and ventral; at the junction of the two the cuticle projects distally onto the nail surface. The lateral nail folds are in continuity with the skin on the sides of the digit laterally, and medially they are joined by the nail bed.

The nail matrix (Figure 4.1) can be subdi-

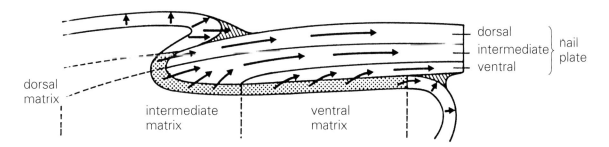

Figure 4.1

Nail matrix compartments and their contribution to the nail plate. The intermediate (proximal) matrix produces the thickest layer (approximately two-thirds of the whole).

vided into dorsal and intermediate sections, the latter underlying the nail plate to the distal border of the lunula; some texts prefer the terms proximal and distal matrix respectively. It is now generally considered that the nail bed contributes to the deep surface of the nail plate (ventral matrix), though this deep component plays little part in the functional integrity of the nail plate in its distal part. At the point of separation of the nail plate from the nail bed, the proximal part of the hyponychium may be modified as the solehorn. Beyond the solehorn region the hyponychium terminates at the distal nail groove; the tip of the digit beyond this ridge assumes the structure of the epidermis elsewhere.

When the attached nail plate is viewed from above several distinct areas may be visible; the proximal lunule and the larger pink zone. On close examination two further distal zones can often be identified, the distal yellowish-white margin and immediately proximal to this the onychodermal band. This is a barely perceptible narrow transverse band 0.5–1.5 mm wide. The exact anatomical basis for the onychodermal (onychocorneal) band is not known but it appears to have a different blood supply than the main body of the nail bed; if the tip of the digit is pressed firmly, the band and an area just proximal to it blanch, and if the pressure is repeated several times the band reddens.

Proximal nail fold

The proximal nail fold is similar in structure to the adjacent skin but is normally devoid of dermatoglyphic markings and pilosebaceous glands. From the distal area of the proximal nail fold the cuticle reflects onto the surface of the nail plate; it is composed of modified stratum corneum and serves to protect the structures at the base of the nail, particularly the germinative matrix, from environmental insults such as irritants, allergens and bacterial

and fungal pathogens. *Nail matrix* (intermediate and dorsal; syn. proximal and distal respectively) is the area which produces the major part of the nail plate. As in the epidermis of the skin, the matrix possesses a dividing basal layer producing keratinocytes which differentiate, harden, die and contribute to the nail plate, which is thus analogous to the epidermal stratum corneum. The nail matrix keratinocytes mature and keratinize without kerato-hyalin (granular layer) formation. Apart from this, the detailed cytological changes seen in the matrix epithelium under the electron microscopy are essentially the same as in the epidermis.

The nail matrix contains melanocytes in the lowest two cell layers and these donate pigment to keratinocytes. Under normal circumstances pigment is not visible in the nail plate of white Caucasoid individuals but many Afro-Caribbean subjects show patchy melanogenesis as linear longitudinal pigmented bands. *The nail bed* consists of an epidermal part (ventral matrix) and the underlying dermis closely apposed to the periosteum of the distal phalanx. There is no subcutaneous fat in the nail bed although scattered dermal fat cells may be visible microscopically.

The nail bed epidermal layer (ventral matrix) is usually no more than two or three cells thick, and the transitional zone from living keratinocyte to dead ventral nail plate cell is abrupt, occurring in the space of one horizontal cell layer. As the cells differentiate they are incorporated into the ventral surface of the nail plate and move distally with this layer.

The nail bed dermal collagen is mainly orientated vertically, being directly attached to phalangeal periosteum and the epidermal basal lamina. Within the connective tissue network lie blood vessels, lymphatics, a fine network of elastic fibres and scattered fat cells; at the distal margin, eccrine sweat glands have been seen. The nail plate (Figure 4.1) is made of three horizontal layers; a thin dorsal lamina, the thicker intermediate lamina and a ventral layer from the nail bed. Microscopically, it is composed of flattened squamous cells closely apposed to each other. In older age groups, acidophilic masses are occasionally seen, the so-called pertinax bodies.

The hardness of nail is mainly due to the high sulphur matrix protein, which contrasts with the relatively soft keratin of the epidermis. The normal curvature of the nail relates to the shape of the underlying phalangeal bone to which the nail plate is directly bonded via the vertical connective tissue attached between the subungual epithelium and the periosteum.

There is a rich arterial blood supply to the nail bed and matrix derived from paired digital arteries. The main supply passes into the pulp space of the distal phalanx before reaching the dorsum of the digit. An accessory supply arises further back on the digit and does not enter the pulp space. There are two main arterial arches (proximal and distal) supplying the nail bed and matrix, formed from anastomoses of the branches of the digital arteries. In the event of damage to the main supply in the pulp space, such as may occur with infection of scleroderma, there may be sufficient blood from the accessory vessels to permit normal growth of the nail.

There is a capillary loop system to the whole of the nail fold, but the loops to the roof and matrix are flatter than those below the exposed nail. There are many arteriovenous anastomoses below the nail, glomus bodies, which are concerned with heat regulation. Glomus bodies are important in maintaining acral circulation under cold conditions — arterioles constrict with cold but glomus bodies dilate. The nail bed of fingers and toes contain such bodies (93–501 cm²). Each glomus is an encapsulated oval organ 300 μm long, made up of a tortuous vessel uniting an artery and venule, a nerve supply and a capsule; also within the capsule are many cholinergic muscle cells.

NAIL DYNAMICS

Clinicians used to observing the slow rate of clearance of diseased or damaged nails are apt to view the nail apparatus as a rather inert structure, although it is in fact the centre of very marked kinetic and biochemical activity. Why the nail grows flat, rather than as a heaped up keratinous mass, has generated much thought and discussion. Several factors probably combine to produce a relatively flat nail plate; the orientation of the matrix rete pegs and papillae; the direction of cell differentiation; and the fact that since keratinization takes place within the confines of the nail base, limited by the proximal nail fold dorsally and the terminal phalanx ventrally, the differentiating cells can only move distally and form a flat structure — by the time they leave the confines of the proximal nail fold all the cells are hardened and keratinized. Fingernails grow at approximately 1 cm per 3 months and toenails at one-half of this rate.

In early childhood, the nail plate is relatively thin and may show temporary koilonychia: because of the shape of the matrix, some children show ridges which start laterally by the proximal nail fold and join at a central point just short of the free margin.

Many of the changes seen in old age may occur in younger age groups with impaired arterial blood supply. Elastic tissue changes diffusely affecting the nail bed epidermis are often seen histologically. The whole subungual area in old age may show thickening of blood vessel walls with vascular elastic tissues fragmentation. Pertinax bodies are often seen in the nail plate; they are probably remnants of nuclei of keratinocytes. Nail growth is inversely proportional to age; related to this slower growth, corneocytes are larger in old age.

The nail plate becomes paler, dull and opaque with advancing years and white nails similar to those seen in cirrhosis, uraemia and hypoalbuminaemia may be seen in normal subjects.

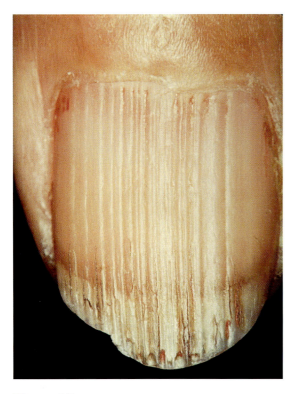

Figure 4.2

Ridged nail, seen increasingly with advancing age.

Longitudinal ridging is present to some degree in most people after 50 years of age and this may give a 'sausage links' appearance.

Foot function

When considering toenail problems, it is of great importance to take a full view of the whole foot. All too often, practitioners treat the nail and foot as static anatomical structures when commonly problems arise as a result of their dynamic functions.

Looking at possible external and locomotor precursors of nail disease, there are distinct differences between fingernails and toenails which need to be considered. Being an appendage to the foot, the nail is often contained in footwear for long periods of time and may be subjected to the forces generated during normal locomotion. Detective work is often needed to highlight causative factors of toenail pathology. These include:

- foot function
- foot shape
- footwear
- occupation and other factors.

In simple terms, the human foot has evolved to carry out a specific function — to assist smooth and efficient locomotion. In undertaking this task the foot has developed the ability to alter its structure and as a consequence, its function within a single footstep. To understand this we must briefly look at the normal gait cycle (see page 23).

Many abnormal foot functions can upset the sequence of supination — pronation — resupination. In terms of toenail pathology, these primarily occur around the propulsive phase of the gait cycle. If for any reason the foot has been unable to supinate to an adequate degree, there may not be adequate rigidity and propulsion occurs on a 'flexible' foot. The result of this is that major forces may be dissipated through the forefoot, and repeated many hundreds of times a day, this can have adverse effects on the digital area, especially when interacting with footwear. If a foot is pronating excessively on propulsion, the foot will elongate (as part of pronation) so the distal area will be subject to trauma if the footwear is inadequate in length. Control of the excessive pronation may be obtained by way of prescribed orthoses in footwear.

Foot shape

Foot shape is of major importance when considering precursors to toenail disease.

be congenital or acquired. Commonly seen is the foot with the second toe slightly longer than the first. This can lead to the longer toe suffering increased trauma from the end of a shoe or stubbing and secondary onychomycosis. Longer toes may suffer trauma in the shoe leading to subungual haematoma and consequent long term changes in the nail structure. Other types of digital deformities may also predispose to pathology of the nail. Neurological disturbances within the lower limb as a result of diabetes, paresis or other disorders can lead to changes in muscular tone within the leg. Spasticity or atrophy may lead to imbalances between dorsiflexors and plantar flexors of the foot which, in turn, result in digital deformities and nail distortion; the latter will vary in relation to the specific paralysis or orthopaedic change.

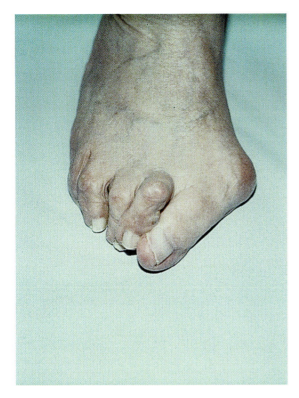

Figure 4.3
Hallux abductovalgus.

Within any population there is a great variation in foot shape and it is important to bear in mind that foot shape will change with age and the effects of disease. A good example is *hallux abductovalgus* (Figure 4.3) — at a young age all that may be apparent is slight first metatarsal head enlargement, but within a few years one sees the gradual deviation of the hallux laterally often under-riding the second toe, forcing it into the upper of a shoe. Such changes in foot shape will inevitably affect foot and nail function. Commonly, medial rotation of the toe accompanied by its abduction towards the second toe, causes the flesh around the nail edge to roll over the nail plate — a precursor to the development of ingrowing toenails.

Problems with the lesser digits can also adversely affect the nail apparatus. These can

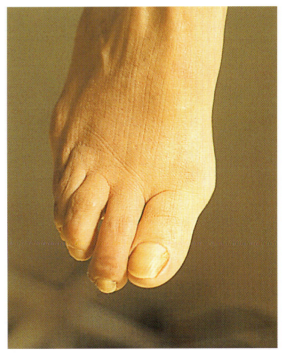

Figure 4.4
Long second toe: nail may be selectively subjected to traumatic factors.

Footwear

Footwear is most often overlooked as a causative or contributory factor in nail disease (Figures 4.5–4.7). When questioned about their footwear, patients will often state that their shoes feel comfortable — 'its just my toenail that hurts when I wear them'. Nail pathology from shoes can be due to many factors:

- poor fitting of footwear
- inadequate footwear design or construction
- excessive wear to shoes.

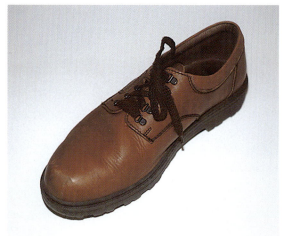

Figure 4.7
Shoe with a seamless front — a good design feature that prevents trauma to digits.

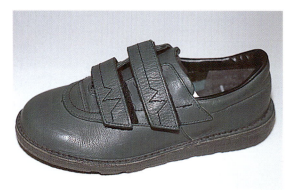

Figure 4.5
Shoe with velcro straps (alternative to lace-ups).

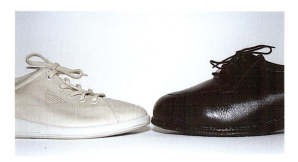

Figure 4.6
Shoes positioned tip to tip, highlighting different depths as a possible contribution to nail problems.

When looking at shoe fitting, areas of prime importance are: *Heel height* — generally if heels are too high, the foot is forced forward into the toe box with every step, traumatizing the anterior part of the foot, especially around the nail apparatus and apices. The higher the heel, the more damage is likely to occur. *Lack of suitable fastening* — a foot in a shoe without adequate fastening suffers in that the foot is free to move unrestrained in the shoe and inevitably (as with high heels) it tends to slip forward into the toe box region of the shoe, traumatizing the distal aspect including the nails. *Poor toe box design* — in order to restrict rubbing and other trauma to the forefoot and nails, a good toe box is a vital feature. Adequate depth and width ensure that no undue pressure is placed on the digital areas; allied with a suitable fastening, this ensures that the foot stays well back from the tip of the shoe and into the heel. One can often see the effects of this when toe outlines are visible from the outside of the shoe. When looking at toenail problems it is wise to feel inside the upper of the shoe; one may often feel a dent or tear in the inner lining of the shoe corresponding to the affected digit. Other clues can be given by the nail itself. A nail with unusual pigmentation may have acquired this from rubbing on the leather of new shoes. More commonly though, a single toenail with a very 'polished' sheen to it can be the result of continuous rubbing on the soft lining of an upper of a shoe. Shoes which are too long or without a fastening can often lead to increased nail trauma as to compensate for the excessive movement, toes become clawed to maintain ground contact and increase stability.

When looking at causative factors of nail problems one must always take into account patients' circumstances. The amount of time a person spends on their feet may affect the severity of the nail problem. Moreover, the footwear worn for these periods of time will be crucial. Occupational footwear can be notorious for precipitating such problems.

Occlusive type footwear worn for long periods of time can lead to retention of excessive perspiration. This may predispose to infection which may go on to affect the nail and surrounding tissues. This is often seen in manual workers who spend long periods of time in rubber or plastic boots or similar footwear: occlusive footwear also contributes to juvenile plantar dermatosis (page 100).

The transportation and construction industries provide the highest incidence of foot injuries. Since the introduction of steel toe cap shoes these have reduced, but even these are not without their problems. The rigidity of the toe box has meant that incorrectly fitting boots have lead to toe and nail injuries as a result of their design.

It is thus very important when considering toenail diseases, be they primary and localized, or due to some more general skin or systemic disease, to consider the nails in relation to toe and foot function in general — in every case! For example even psoriasis affecting all 20 nails may require podiatric and footwear attention to maintain foot function as a unit (Figure 4.8).

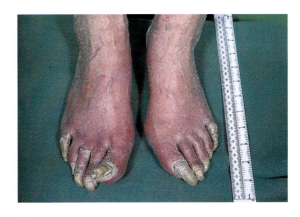

Figure 4.8

Psoriasis. This patient had psoriatic plaques and scalp lesions. The feet show much hyperkeratotic change due to friction and pressure (Koebner phenomenon).

Practitioners all too often treat the nail and foot as static anatomical structures when common problems frequently arise as a result of their dynamic functions.

It is pertinent in this context to consider in more detail the most common orthopaedic and traumatic disorders that may lead to nail disorders or worsen the effects of primary nail diseases from other causes.

Hallux abductovalgus

This is a progressive deviation of the big toe laterally, often accompanied by valgus rotation of the toe (Figure 4.3). As the big toe deviates, a medial prominence develops on the first metatarsal head and becomes inflamed as it rubs on footwear. The second digit frequently overrides the deviating big toe or develops a hammer deformity. The condition occurs most commonly in women and usually shows a familial pattern. The exact aetiology is

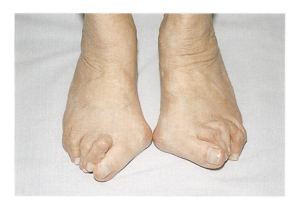

Figure 4.9
Hallux abductovalgus. Rotation of the digit can place extra pressure around the nail when walking.

unknown. Most frequently poor footwear can be implicated, although studies have shown the existence of hallux abductovalgus in unshod races. Also excessively pronated feet have been highlighted as a predisposing factor; inflammatory joint diseases appear to accelerate its development. This disorder places great stresses on the nail apparatus of the great toe and adjacent nails (Figure 4.9) which frequently become distorted, thickened onychogryphotic or ingrown. Treatment of the condition depends on the symptoms, primary care being direct relief or discomfort. Where excessive pronation coexists, the use of orthoses may give relief of symptoms. Surgery for hallux valgus is indicated where severe deformity develops on or when pain relief is not achieved with conservative methods. The effectiveness of night splints to straighten the big toe is questionable.

Hallux limitus and rigidus

Hallux limitus and rigidus are common conditions of the first toe where there is either reduced or total loss of dorsiflexion at the metatarsophalangeal joint. The deformity is often accompanied by dorsal enlargement of the first metatarsal head and hyperextension of the big toe. Clinically, it is most frequent in men; morning pain which often wears off during the day is the main complaint: it is aggravated by prolonged standing or activity. Alteration of the normal gait pattern to alleviate the pain may often result in secondary lesions such as plantar corns and callosities; and irregular thickening of the big toenail, secondary onychomycosis and ingrowing nail.

In normal function the range of motion of the first metatarsophalangeal joint should be sufficient for heel list and toe dorsiflexion. If this is limited, body weight is forced through the interphalangeal joint of the big toe causing hyperextension of the toe and hypertrophy of the nail, leaving them prone to damage from shallow footwear. The primary cause of the disorder is unknown but theories include trauma setting up a localized osteoarthritis in the joint, a long first metatarsal, or excessively pronated foot type causing restriction of normal movement of the foot.

Treatment of the condition is by symptomatic relief. Elimination of aggravating factors may help, i.e. footwear modification/advice. Insoles and orthoses are of benefit to realign the foot and redistribute weight bearing away from the painful joint and nail. In acute painful stages of the disease, immobilization, by way of strapping of the toe, may be of benefit.

Lesser toe deformities

The stability and function of the digit is easily altered by abnormal foot function (excessive pronation and supination). Some of the more common digital deformities are:

- Clawing or retraction of toes arises most commonly as the result of inflammatory joint disease or supinated foot types. Plantar flexion of the metatarsals gives a mechanical advantage to the long extensor tendons of the foot, which inevitably pull the toes into dorsal retraction. Consequently, this causes rubbing on footwear and hyperkeratoses develop on the toes. Moreover, excessive weight is borne on the now prominent metatarsal heads, because digital weight bearing is diminished, leading to metatarsalgia

- Adductovarus deformity of the lesser toes is thought to be a result of excessive pronation, flattening the arch and altering the angle of pull of the long flexor tendons. Hyperkeratotic lesions are common on the apices of these toes
- Hammer toe deformity is often a secondary effect seen with hallux abductovalgus; rarely is it a congenital deformity.

All these digital deformities are commonly associated with irregularly thickened and distorted toenails which may mimic onychomycosis.

Nail changes

Nail deformity often occurs as an end result of digital deformity compounded by poorly fitting footwear, or trauma, or of altered foot shape resulting from other problems such as hallux abductovalgus.

Subungual haematoma

This common condition occurs as a result of acute trauma to the nail plate from injury, poorly fitting footwear or after long distance running (e.g. marathons) (Figure 4.10). Haemorrhage leads to the accumulation of

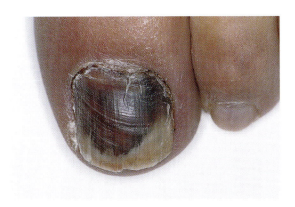

Figure 4.10
Subungual haematoma due to rubbing against a poorly fitting shoe.

blood under the nail plate, forcing its separation from the nail bed which causes pain. Athletes in 'stamina' sports often get degrees of painless subungual haemorrhage. Prompt release of acute haematoma (within 24 hours) by piercing the nail plate improves the chances of retaining the nail and affords pain relief. Lesions resembling subungual haematoma without a history of trauma should be monitored and regarded with suspicion because, rarely, the condition may mimic subungual melanoma.

Onychauxis and onychogryphosis

Onychauxis is a thickening of the entire nail plate. Most commonly observed in the big toe, the condition is often the result of trauma (repeated or single) to the nail; skin disease, such as psoriasis (Figure 4.8), may also lead to the condition. Digital deformity can accompany the condition. It is more commonly seen in elderly people, and fungal colonization may occur. Onychogryphosis (ram's horn deformity) is a similar affliction, but in this case the nail tends to deviate laterally as it grows (Figures 4.11, 4.12). This is usually the result of trauma (occupational or footwear) or sometimes results from earlier untreated onychomycosis. As the nail thickens, nail care becomes difficult. Podiatric treatment of the affected nails is by reduction of the thickened plate with a nail drill. Total avulsion of the nail plate with phenolization of the nail matrix offers a permanent solution to the problem.

Onychocryptosis: ingrowing toenail

This is the embedding of the lateral toenail edges into the sulci, piercing the flesh, and leading to local paronychia and secondary bacterial infection (Figure 4.13). The condition is most commonly observed in the big toe of physically active young adult men and can result from poor nail cutting technique aggravated by footwear and trauma. Particular nail shapes may be at greater risk of developing the problem. As the embedded nail grows forward, hypergranulation tissue may protrude from the nail sulcus. Isolated occurrences of onychocryptosis may be resolved by conservative removal of the offending spicule and packing the sulcus with cotton wool. Antibiotic cover should be given where secondary bacte-

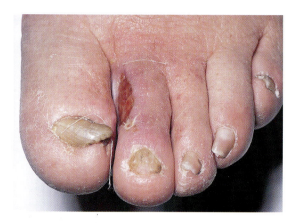

Figure 4.11
Early onychogryphosis (ram's horn deformity).

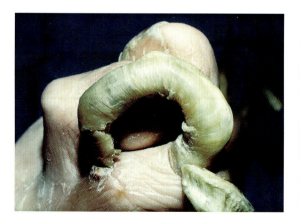

Figure 4.12
Severe onychogryphosis.

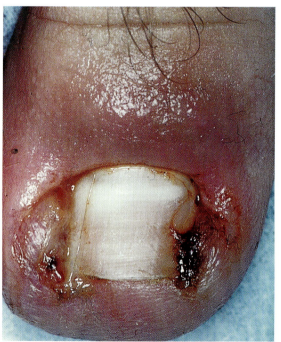

Figure 4.13
Ingrowing toenail (onychocryptosis).

rial infection is suspected. Education is vital to minimize recurrence. If conservative investigation, observation and antiseptic principles have failed, then a simple surgical operation is usually curative. Before proceeding to surgery:

- check footwear — may be cause
- check foot and toe shape, and function
- check for onychomycosis
- check that nail trimming is being carried out correctly
- check the antiseptic or antibiotic treatment if chronic inflammation or infection is present.

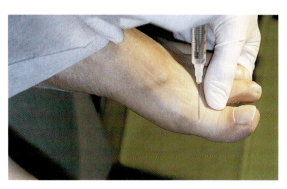

Figures 4.15a
Digital block with anaesthetic.

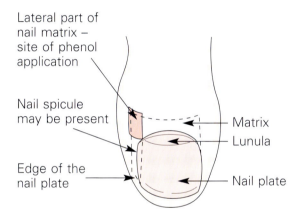

Figure 4.14
Ingrowing toenail showing matrix to be phenolized.

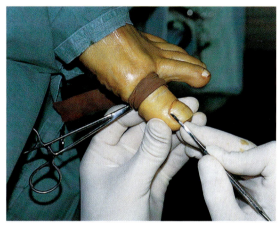

Figure 4.15b
Loosening of the nail from the nail bed using a Black's file.

The surgical procedure involved (Figure 4.14) is minimally invasive and is associated with a low recurrence or regrowth rate. The procedure can involve partial or total ablation of the nail plate (Figures 4.15a-k). Nail ablation may also be indicated for onychogryphosis, involuted nail and onychauxis (thickened toenail).

A local anaesthetic is administered. A digital ring block is performed (see page 143). Figure 4.15a shows a self-aspirating dental-type syringe being used. These are particularly well suited to digital anaesthesia; anaesthetic solution without adrenaline should be used.

The toe is prepared with betadine alcoholic solution and exanguiation of the toe is achieved using an Esmarch bandage (Figure 4.15b). This ensures a bloodless field during the procedure and is necessary to maximize the effect of the phenol when destroying the nail matrix. A Black's file is used to separate the nail plate from the surrounding skin and eponychium.

A Francis nail elevator can be used to free the nail plate from the nail bed (Figure 4.15c).

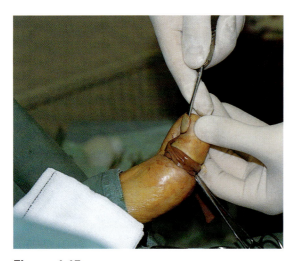

Figure 4.15c

Elevation of the nail.

For a partial nail ablation it is only necessary to free the minimum edge of nail destined for removal. For a total nail ablation, however, the whole nail plate should be separated from the nail bed.

For partial nail ablation a straight section of nail plate is cut using a Thwaite's nipper (Figure 4.15d). It is important to cut as far proximal as possible and to maintain a straight

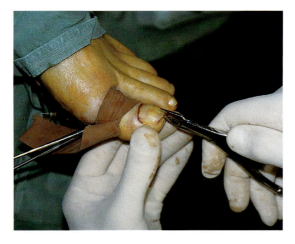

Figure 4.15d

The nail plate is cut using a Thwaite's nipper.

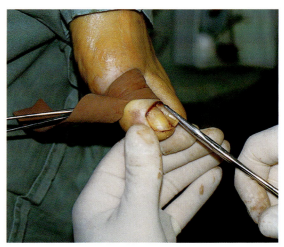

Figure 4.15e

Forceps locking into the nail plate.

cut. Only the minimum section of nail needs to be cut.

Forceps are 'locked' onto the section of nail to be removed and rotated slowly towards the middle of the nail plate (Figure 4.15e). This ensures the complete removal of the offending section of nail plate. It is important to secure the forceps to the most offending section of nail plate as possible. Check the removed section nail for a 'feathery' proximal aspect.

Total nail plate ablation can be achieved similarly by locking forceps onto one edge of the nail plate and rotating towards the midline of the nail plate. Often the nail will come away in one piece.

Prior to phenolization of the exposed nail bed and remaining matrix the surrounding tissues should be masked with petroleum jelly. Figure 4.15f shows sterile petroleum jelly being applied from a tulle-gras dressing (e.g. Bactigras, Jelonet). Care should be taken to prevent the jelly coming into contact with the nail bed and matrix as this will prevent penetration of the phenol.

Phenol is applied to the nail bed and matrix using sterile cotton buds. These can be constructed from sterile orange sticks and

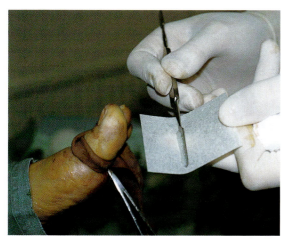

Figure 4.15f

Masking of the surrounding tissue with petro-leum jelly.

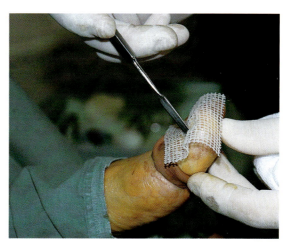

Figure 4.15h

Packing the site with tulle gras.

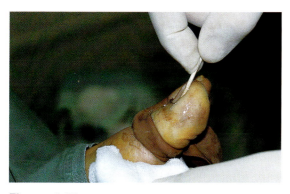

Figure 4.15g

Application of the phenol.

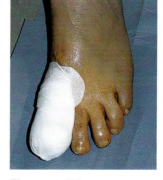

Figure 4.15i

Final post-operative dressing.

cotton wool (Figure 4.15g). Action of phenol can be enhanced by first abrading the target nail bed and matrix with a Black's file. Maximum strength phenol should be used. Phenol crystals will melt when placed in a bottle stood in a cup of hot water, this is an ideal preparation. Do not add hot water to the phenol crystals. Alternatively 85 per cent liquefied phenol can be used. Phenol should be applied for 3 minutes if melted cystalized, or 5-6 minutes if 85 per cent liquefied. Several applications should be worked into the nail bed and matrix during this time.

It is not necessary to 'neutralize' or dilute the phenol at the end of the phenolization time. However, a tulle dressing can be packed into the cavity to protect the finalized tissues (Figure 4.15h). A simple dressing consisting of non-adherent dressing, gauze, tabanid and sticking plaster is placed over the site (Figure 4.15i). The patient is advised to keep the toe dry and clean unto the wound is healed.

Post-operative pain is usually minimal and can normally be controlled with simple analgesics. Healing is delayed by the phenol

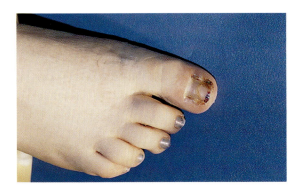

Figure 4.15j

Post-operative appearance of a partial nail avulsion.

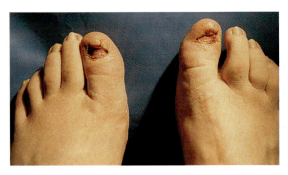

Figure 4.15k

Post-operative appearance of a total nail avulsion.

and it can take up to 6-8 weeks before a complete recovery is achieved. Incidence of regrowth is less than 5 per cent with this technique.

Figure 4.15j shows the post-operative appearance of a partial nail avulsion. Figure 4.15k shows the post-operative appearance of bilateral total nail avulsions.

- the wound will remain moist for 2–3 weeks
- dress regularly until healing is completed.

There are a variety of physical signs that may present with toenail involvement. Many of these may be more obvious in the toes because of traumatic factors: therefore, always examine fingernails in disorders of the toenails!

Splinter haemorrhages

Splinter haemorrhages may be defined as 2–3 mm linear haemorrhages, usually in the longitudinal axis of the nail bed (Figure 4.16). They are normally non-specific phenomena, which, in small number in a single digit, are of no significance. The causes of splinter haemorrhages are as follows:

- idiopathic
- local trauma
- local dermatoses: eczema, psoriasis, onychomycosis, scurvy, pemphigus
- vessel diseases: collagen vascular disease/ Raynaud's phenomenon, septicaemia and septic emboli, blood dyscrasia, hepatitis and cirrhosis.

The mechanism of splinter haemorrhage formation is illustrated in Figure 4.17.

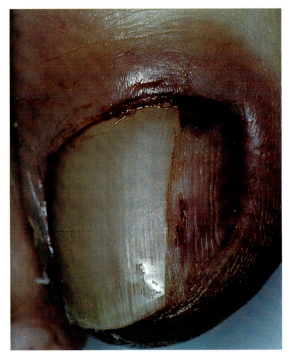

Figure 4.16

Splinter haemorrhage: site in the nail bed.

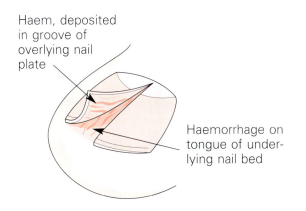

Haem, deposited in groove of overlying nail plate

Haemorrhage on tongue of under-lying nail bed

Figure 4.17
Mechanism of splinter haemorrhage formation.

Pincer deformity; involution

Pincer deformity or involution is caused by trans-verse overcurvature that increases distally (Figure 4.18). This is cosmetically undesirable and occ-asionally painful. In the feet it has been attributed to ill-fitting shoes or distortion of the proximal nail matrix by osteophytes. At all sites it may be due to a subungual exostosis, which should be sought by X-ray. Distal overcurvature may eventually produce loss of nail bed, and funnel or claw formation.

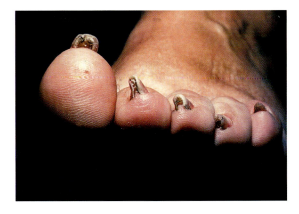

Figure 4.18
Pincer nail deformity.

Hook and claw nails

Hook and claw nails occur when nails grow adhering to the terminal aspect of the digital pulp and curving onto the plantar surface. Often, the little toes are affected due to trauma caused by high-heeled shoes or, in other toes, after fracture of the terminal phalanx. The condition can occasionally be congenital or associated with the nail-patella syndrome.

Nail atrophy

Nail atrophy occurs when there is a reduction in surface area and thickness of the nail, often accompanied by splitting and variable loss (Figures 4.19, 4.20). Pterygium (a ridge of fibrous tissue) may form in some scarring types of nail atrophy. This involves a fibrotic

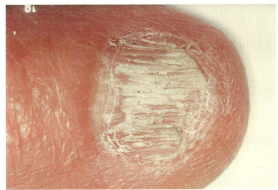

Figure 4.19
Nail atrophy, here due to lichen planus.

extension of the proximal nail fold into the adjacent nail bed in the case of dorsal ptery-gium. Ventral pterygium is a similar process but occurs subungually and is visible distally. Dorsal pterygium will always result in some permanent disfigurement. In routine clinical

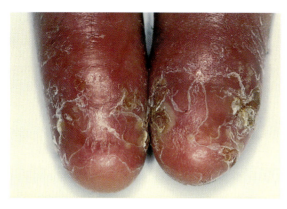

Figure 4.20
Severe nail atrophy, due to erosive lichen planus.

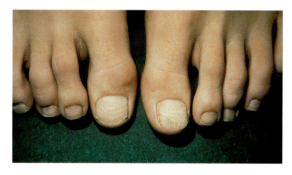

Figure 4.21
Rough nails (trachyonychia): may be idiopathic or due to lichen planus or alopecia areata.

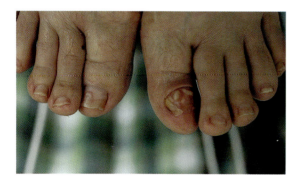

Figure 4.22
Psoriasis: pustular variety with onycholysis of right great toe.

practice lichen planus is the commonest cause though scarring bullous diseases must be considered.

Rough nails — trachyonychia

In trachyonychia there is a roughness of the nail surface as if it had been longitudinally rubbed with sandpaper (Figure 4.21). In more extreme forms the nail becomes brittle and fragments at the free edge. There are several causes of rough nails — the most common is an idiopathic 20-nail dystrophy (which may not always involve all 20 nails). This has a variable associated with autoimmune disorders, most particularly lichen planus and alopecia areata. Complete or partial resolution is likely in children, but not always in adults.

Onycholysis

Onycholysis is a separation of the nail from the nail bed at the distal or lateral margins (Figure 4.22). The split is made apparent by a change in the normal pink colour seen through the nail. Pus, air and shed squames give a yellow appearance. Infection with pseudomonas species gives a green hue, and blood gives a red to brown or black colour. A serum-like exudate containing glycoproteins produces an 'oily spot' or 'salmon patch' as seen in psoriasis. By far the most common causes of onycholysis are psoriasis, fungus/candida species, and trauma.

Pachyonychia

A normal fingernail is about 0.5 mm thick and a toenail twice this. Hyperkeratosis of the nail bed may cause apparent thickening, whereas changes in the matrix result in real thickening (Figure 4.23). Often the two types of pachyonychia occur together. In onychogryphosis, thickening of the nail is due to lack of cutting and distortion due to ill-fitting footwear and/or hallux valgus. This usually involved the great toe of the elderly and is occasionally related to vascular abnormalities in the affected limb.

Leuconychia

True leuconychia is an abnormality which originates in the matrix; the nail appears white (Figure 4.24). It may take any of four forms: the entire nail, as longitudinal or transverse lines, or as isolated white patches. Pseudoleuconychia is a white nail caused by disease outside the matrix, e.g. onychomycosis. Apparent leuconychia is a spurious whiteness due to changes in subungual tissues. The causes of these conditions include psoriasis, dermatitis, various metabolic diseases, onychomycosis, anaemia, cirrhosis and renal disease.

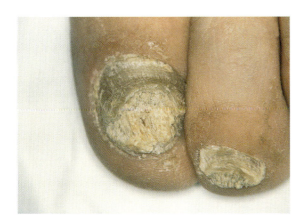

Figure 4.23
Pachyonychia: traumatic, with secondary fungal invasion.

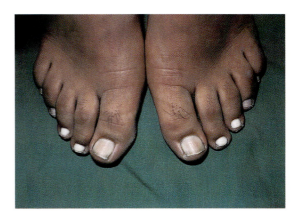

Figure 4.24
Congenital leuconychia.

Melanonychia

Melanonychia is a black or brown discolouration of the nail, usually longitudinal (Figures 4.25–4.29). Biological melanonychia is due to either haem or melanin on the undersurface of the nail, or in the nail itself. Artefactual melanonychia is produced by the action of exogenous pigments, on the outer surface. Clinically, the critical decision is whether or not the pigment derives from a malignant melanoma. On the foot such tumour change is almost always on the great toe. The causes of melanonychia include:

* idiopathic, including pigmented naevi
* racial (almost 100 per cent) of middle-aged Afro-Caribbeans)
* trauma
* onychomycosis
* malignant melanoma
* bacterial infection
* benign melanocytic lesion, hypoadrenalism
* Laugier–Hunziker syndrome (with buccal pigmentation)
* lichen planus.

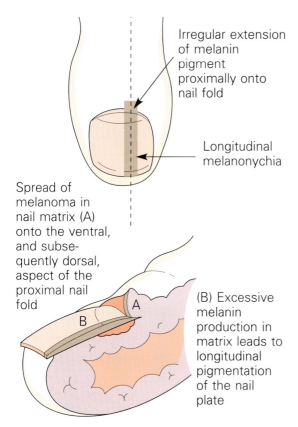

Irregular extension of melanin pigment proximally onto nail fold

Longitudinal melanonychia

Spread of melanoma in nail matrix (A) onto the ventral, and subsequently dorsal, aspect of the proximal nail fold

(B) Excessive melanin production in matrix leads to longitudinal pigmentation of the nail plate

Figure 4.25
Origin of pigment in malignant melanoma of the nail unit.

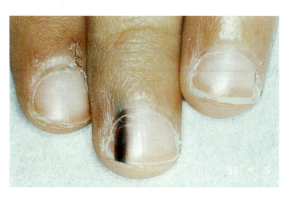

Figure 4.26
Linear melanonychia: pigmented naevus.

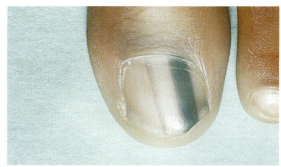

Figure 4.27
Linear melanonychia: normal Afro-Caribbean nails.

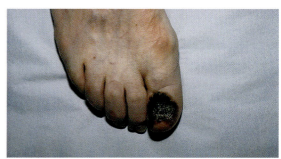

Figure 4.28
Malignant melanoma.

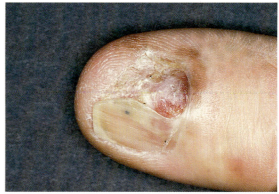

Figure 4.29
Malignant melanoma: pigment spreading away from nail (Hutchinson's sign).

It is often necessary to make the distinction between a melanocytic lesion and a haematoma. Furthermore, no practitioner can be criticized for referring any melanonychia because morbidity due to subungual melanoma is high, even with early diagnosis. The first observation should be the site of origin of the pigment. Melanomas have only been identified arising from the matrix (i.e. from the lunula or more proximally). Haematomas may develop anywhere. A history of trauma does not help unless it is very definite. The most valuable difference in the history is that a haematoma will grow out with the nail, unlike a melanoma. The situation is less clear if the digit is subject to repeated trauma so that a new haematoma is being constantly produced and masks the growing out appearance. Equally, the diagnosis is made more difficult if the haematoma is only partly attributable to trauma and there is an underlying lesion that bleeds easily. Consequently, a bore hole in the nail to identify blood is not sufficient to exclude a neoplasm. A persistent melanonychia that fails to grow out requires an expert opinion, which will usually involve biopsy. Additional factors that make a melanoma more likely are:

- only one digit involved
- spread of the pigment onto the proximal nail fold (Hutchinson's sign)
- rapidly progressive widening of the streak with blurred borders
- age over 50 years
- darkening of the longitudinal streak.

Onychomycosis

Onychomycosis (Figures 4.30, 4.31a–e) is a fungal infection of the nail apparatus. This may involve the nail bed, matrix and plate, either in isolation or together. The main pathogen is trichophyton species, but scopularopsis brevicaulis is sometimes isolated, typically when

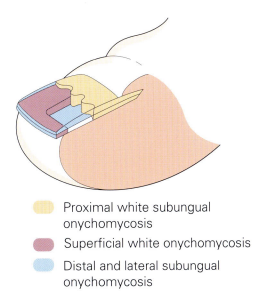

■ Proximal white subungual onychomycosis

■ Superficial white onychomycosis

■ Distal and lateral subungual onychomycosis

Total dystrophic onychomycosis occurs when all three sites are involved

Figure 4.30
Patterns of fungal nail infection.

there is a cloudy infection of half of one great toe. Yeast (candida albicans) and pseudomonas infections may occur alone or in association with a fungus. Pseudomonas infections cause a characteristic green colour. The terminology of the location of a fungal infection is described in Figure 4.30.

Diagnosis: nail clippings and subungual scrapings

Part of the sample can be examined under the microscopy after soaking in 20–30 per cent potassium hydroxide solution to dissolve the keratin. The rest should be sent for microbiology. Specimens survive well in the post, and the chance of an accurate result is increased if the nail specimen exceeds 3 mm in width.

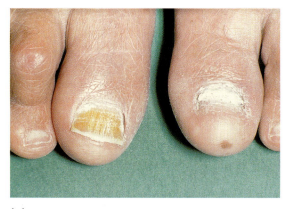

(a)

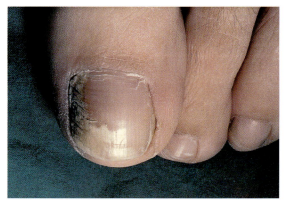

(b)

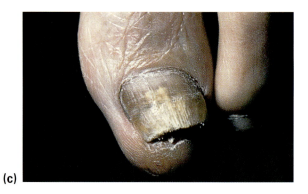

(c)

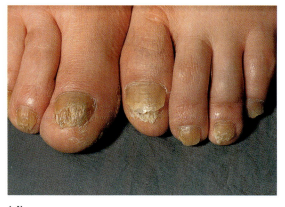

(d)

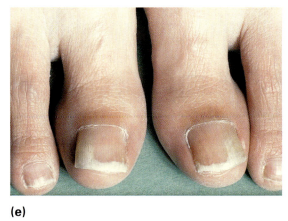

(e)

Figure 4.31
(a–e) Onychomycosis.

Nail biopsy

This is not routinely recommended. To have fungi identified by a pathologist a periodic acid-Schiff (PAS) stain must be requested (Figure 4.32). It can be performed on an isolated piece

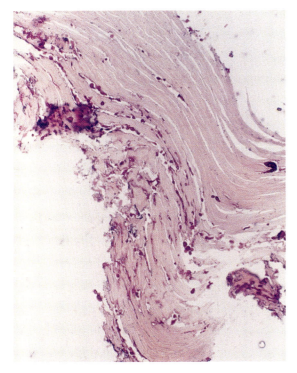

Figure 4.32
Red fungal elements seen: nail tissue stained with periodic acid-Schiff (PAS).

of nail and associated subungual material. The specimen should not be a fragment, but a substantial sample of nail and underlying tissue, e.g. 3 mm punch biopsy. A biopsy is most helpful if the differential of psoriasis or another dermatosis is being considered. In such cases it is necessary that nail and underlying tissue be biopsied. This has the potential for scarring and is best performed by a dermatologist. It is important to recognize that the isolation of

fungus from a dystrophic nail does not prove that it is the cause of the dystrophy. An established dystrophy is susceptible to colonization by fungus, which may further damage the nail. This can sometimes account for the lack of complete resolution of a presumed onychomycosis after appropriate treatment. Equally, the presence of a fungus is not fully excluded by negative microbiology, as effective trial of therapy can show in such cases.

Systemic

Terbinafine is licensed for use in a 6 week course for the treatment of toenail onychomycosis — for a 12–24 week course. Trials suggest that the cure rate is around 80 per cent with only a modest relapse rate in the first year. The drug has relatively few side effects, the most frequently reported complaint being temporary loss of taste. It is not clear how long the drug remains in fat and how this affects advice to women who may subsequently want to become pregnant. The current recommendation is that pregnancy is avoided within 6 months of the last dose. Short treatments are possible.

Itraconazole may give similar results in up to 6 months, although trials of shorter courses show that pulsed therapy, one week in each 4 week period for 4–6 pulses is adequate. These figures may soon be revised, because of the suggestion that the drug may remain active for up to 6 months following a 1 month course. Itraconazole is effective against candida species, whereas oral terbinafine is not so in clinical terms. Both drugs are considerably more expensive than griseofulvin.

Griseofulvin has the advantage of being cheap and of known safety in long courses and in children. It has a higher incidence of side effects, such as gastrointestinal upset and rashes. It is needed for 12–18 months for toenails. The exact duration should be 1 month longer than that needed to ensure clinical clearance; cure is only obtained in a minority of those treated. Griseofulvin is of no use against candida species. In combination therapy, the transungual delivery systems may well bring new life to this old systemic drug, with respect to the shortened duration of treatment and an improved rate of cure. There is sometimes an argument for combining the topical and systemic therapies if previous experience has shown that monotherapy in a particular patient has been unsuccessful. In patients with frequent relapses it has also been suggested that prophylactic use of one of the antifungal nail lacquers may keep the nail disease-free.

Complete surgical avulsion is not usually recommended, because of the potential post-operative complications of bacterial infection and distal ingrowing. These problems are often avoided by removal of only part of the nail by chemical avulsion. Daily applications of 40 per cent urea paste under a dressing will cause keratinolysis and hence detachment of diseased nail over 10–14 days. In this soft state it can be easily pared away. This will increase the efficacy of topical antifungals.

Relapse is common, particularly if preventive measures such as appropriate footwear is not worn. It is important to treat tinea pedis thoroughly as it may otherwise promote onychomycosis.

Psoriasis

Nail features in psoriasis (Figures 4.8, 4.22) include pitting, thickening, onycholysis, dis-colouration, oily spots, splinter haemorrhages, paronychia and pustulation. Psoriasis almost always affects finger and toe nails together if nails are involved.

Periungual and subungual warts

Human papillomavirus infection of the periungual skin and nail apparatus causes periungual and subungual warts (Figures 4.33, 4.34). The diagnosis is usually obvious by the appearance and association with warts elsewhere. Paring the surface may give the characteristic pinpoint bleeding seen in all warts.

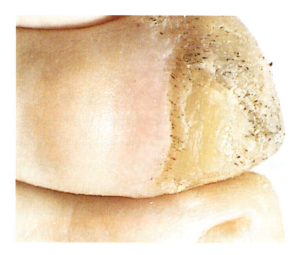

Figure 4.33
Periungual wart causing nail thickening.

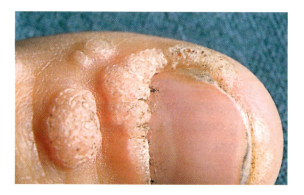

Figure 4.34
Periungual warts in a child, provoked by finger biting.

Warts beneath the nail should be exposed for assessment. They may reflect an underlying bony exostosis, which can be revealed by X-ray. Long-standing, atypical warts occasionally turn out to be a squamous cell carcinoma and therefore warrant biopsy particularly in middle-aged or older patients.

Warts will eventually disappear without treatment, although they can persist longer in the periungual skin and nail apparatus than those at other sites. This may reflect the isomorphic response in which trauma provokes a continuation of the disease.

Salicylic acid treatment is often unsuccessful and can be messy. Great emphasis must be laid upon the correct use of the preparations, which can contain up to 50 per cent salicylic acid in an ointment base, of 17 per cent as a collodion. It is essential that the patient soak and abrade the wart daily before reapplication. Success may be maximized by asking the patient to commence treatment under the supervision of the practice nurse.

Treatment with liquid nitrogen may be painful and should rarely be used in children without topical or injected local anaesthesia. There is little published evidence to suggest that it is more effective than properly applied salicylic acid. There is a potential for scarring the matrix with aggressive freezing. To minimize this, some practitioners use an oblique jet from the gun rather than direct it straight down upon the wart. It is important to use judgement to avoid distress caused by over-treatment. Pain and erythema may be reduced by a single application of very potent steroid. The treatment should be repeated at 3–4 weeks; if the patient is able to use salicylic acid preparations in the meantime, the success rate may be higher.

Bleomycin therapy is occasionally used in hospitals. It should not be used in general practice. It is cytotoxic and is painful when injected directly into the wart. If it is used around the matrix, scarring nail dystrophy may result. It is reserved for particularly troublesome warts, usually in immunosuppressed patients.

As a rule, surgery should be avoided. At the proximal nail fold there is a risk of scarring, making this an undesirable therapy. Subungual or lateral nail fold warts may respond successfully to curettage, but this should be performed with care.

Lichen planus

Lichen planus (Figure 4.35) characteristically affects the skin in the form of flat-topped violaceous papules, with white (Wickham's) striae of mucosal surfaces. It can affect the scalp and axillae to produce a scarring alopecia; and also the nails occasionally without other sites being affected.

The nail changes of lichen planus cover a wide range of appearances and occur in 10 per cent of those with skin involvement. In this 10 per cent the diagnosis is relatively easy. Otherwise, diagnosis is based upon clinical judgement of histology of a longitudinal nail biopsy. If biopsy is made, it should be done early by a dermatologist to prevent characteristic features being replaced by scar tissue. The mildest, non-specific features may be longitu-

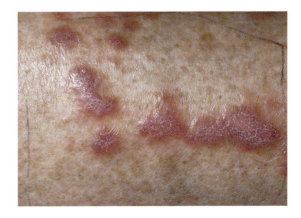

Figure 4.35

Lichen planus: dull–red lesions with surface white striae.

dinal ridges or depressions and occasionally pitting. A more global atrophy of the nail matrix may produce nail fragility and a sandpapered appearance, sometimes with koilonychia. This can affect just a few, or all the nails. More aggressive still is the atrophy that combines with scarring of the matrix and proximal nail fold. This results in pterygium formation, in which the nail may split longitudinally and be all or partly lost, leaving a fibrotic, atrophic nail bed. The condition occurs in children as well as in adults.

Glomus tumour

Glomus tumours are benign and normally occur in 30–50 year olds. When they do so, the tumour is only a few millimetres in diameter and usually gives a substantial amount of pain on pressure and changes in temperature. If the nail bed is involved without impinging on the matrix, there may be very little to see or just a longitudinal pink line through the nail. When the matrix is involved there is a secondary longitudinal nail dystrophy or split. The split may run the entire length of the nail or it may be present as a nick at the distal end of a groove. Excision of the tumour is usually necessary on clinical grounds.

Myxoid cyst

Myxoid cyst (Figure 4.36) most commonly occurs around the proximal nail fold. Transillumination shows a cystic quality. Myxoid cysts are painless. Pressure on the matrix can cause a longitudinal depression in the nail. The overlying proximal nail fold may become verrucous or ulcerated. The adjacent interphalangeal joint often has osteoarthritis and Heberden's nodes. The cyst may repre-

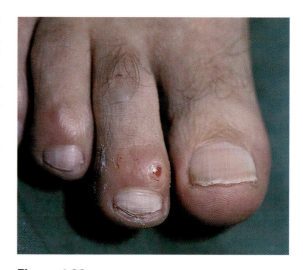

Figure 4.36
Digital myxoid cyst.

sent a ganglion in continuity with this joint. Treatment is best performed by those experienced in dealing with this disease. Methods include plastic surgery, cryosurgery or the cautious injection of 0.1 ml of the sclerosant, 1 per cent sodium tetradecyl sulphate, once a month for 3 months after evacuation of the mucoid content.

Fibroma

Fibromas may occur in the presence or absence of tuberous sclerosis. They are benign tumours, usually seen extending from beneath the proximal or lateral nail fold onto the dorsal aspect of the nail plate. If they are solely ventral to the nail plate, they may appear as a longitudinal subungual red line with minimal symptoms. Emerging at the free edge, or lying on the nail plate, the smooth, firm morphology of these tumours is characteristic.

A variant of fibroma may appear as a 'garlic clove' tumour, often with a small pedicle. This resembles the bulb, with many small fibromas pressed together. Fibromas can be removed surgically, but it is usually necessary to reflect the nail fold to ensure extirpation of the source of the lesion.

Koenen's tumours are fibromas (Figure 4.37). They develop in adolescents with tuberous sclerosis. They are benign and not painful. They can be excized at the base, which may require reflection of the proximal nail fold.

Subungual exostoses

Subungual exostoses (Figure 4.38a, b) are painful and are usually sited in the great toe or thumb of a young adult. They arise beneath the distal nail and cause it to lift up. The exostosis is revealed by X-ray, and treatment is by surgical removal. In the elderly, hyperostosis may contribute to pincer nail formation, especially in the great toe.

Bowen's disease and squamous cell carcinoma

Both Bowen's disease and squamous cell carcinoma can occur around the nail unit and be present many years before the diagnosis is made. They may be eczematous, warty, weeping or resembling paronychia, and so may provide lots of reasons to delay a diagnostic biopsy. When faced with an atypical lesion that does not get better after more than 6 months of appropriate treatment, a biopsy should always be performed. Surgical excision or Moh's chemosurgery are the most common definitive treatments.

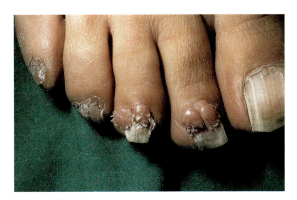

Figure 4.37
Periungual fibromas: Koenen's tumours.

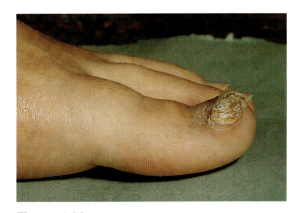

Figure 4.38a
Subungual exostosis.

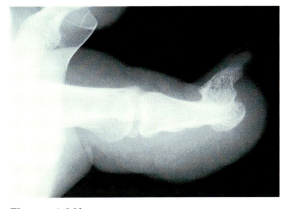

Figure 4.38b
Subungual exostosis: X-ray changes.

5 Aspects of skin therapeutics

INTRODUCTION
TOPICAL AND ORAL TREATMENTS
PHYSICAL AND SURGICAL TREATMENTS

INTRODUCTION

Very specific medical and physical therapies are described in appropriate sections. In this chapter general aspects of some topical and oral treatments are considered together with some surgical treatment that potentially bestride both podiatry and dermatology practice.

TOPICAL AND ORAL TREATMENTS

There are a number of therapeutic agents which are predominantly used in the treatment of skin diseases. It is important that one has some knowledge of these treatments. As the skin is the most accessible organ of the body, many common drugs are used topically and the pharmacological principles of topical therapy are rarely taught to medical students and associated health professionals.

In deciding whether topical or oral treatment should be used, the following points should be remembered. If the lesion is dermal rather than epidermal, then topical measures will be of little or no use. Clinically, a lesion is dermal and not epidermal if there is no scaling, crusting or weeping of the skin surface. Topical measures are of little value in dermal disorders for two reasons. Firstly, if the epidermis is intact, it is unlikely that a sufficiently high concentration of the drug will penetrate the skin barrier (normal keratin); secondly, if the drug does penetrate the epidermis and reaches the dermis, it is then absorbed into the tissue fluid and bloodstream, and is rapidly diluted at the site where it is expected to act. If the lesion is mainly or partly epidermal, then topical preparations are indicated. Topical preparations are likely to be more effective in these cases because the epidermal barrier has been destroyed by the disease process and, as the epidermis has no blood vessels, systemically administered drugs can only reach the epidermal cells by diffusion through cells and intercellular fluid.

Thus, a higher concentration of the drug is often obtained in the epidermis by topical rather than systemic administration. The advantage of topically applied drugs compared with those systemically administered is that the disease organ is specifically treated while the rest of the body is not exposed to the drug (or to only a very small concentration).

Vehicles for topical preparations

Clinicians are often confused because they need to know not only which drug to use for the disorder, but also with which vehicle to administer the drug. Basically, topical preparations can be divided into four groups; solutions; creams; ointments; and pastes:

Solutions

The drug should be used in solution form when the skin is acutely inflamed, as manifested by weeping or exudation from the skin surface. Solutions are also indicated for dermatoses in the intertriginous areas (i.e. where two skin surfaces are in apposition, e.g. groins, axillae and between the toes). It should be noted that solutions evaporate quickly if applied to the skin surface and, thus, the duration of action of the drug on the diseased area is relatively short, perhaps as little as 30 minutes. Therefore, if continuous treatment of the skin surface is required, lotions have to be applied very frequently.

Creams

These are emulsions of either water dispersed in oil or oil dispersed in water. They have a relatively high content of water compared with oil. Clinically, this means they are pleasant and non-greasy to use, and the patients find that they are well absorbed into the skin. A cream should be chosen as the vehicle for a drug in sub-acute conditions, e.g. when there is slight exudation, and in disorders affecting the intertriginous areas. The duration of action of the drug can be expected to be longer than that of a solution, but shorter than that of an ointment, probably around 4–5 hours. Thus, if continuous treatment of diseased skin is required, the cream should be applied every 4–5 hours; this may however vary depending on the active agent.

Ointments

Clinically, these substances are 'greasy'. Chemically, there are three different types: those which are water-soluble; those which emulsify with water; and those which do not mix with water. However, it is their clinical properties that are important. Because these substances are greasy, they should not be used in cases with acute weeping or sub-acute skin disease, or in the intertriginous areas, particularly the groins and under the breasts. The main indication for their use is the presence of 'dry' chronic dermatoses. The duration of action of the drug in an ointment base if longer than that in a cream and in general needs to be applied 2–3 times a day for continuous action of the drug on the skin. As a basic rule, a drug (particularly a steroid) in an ointment base is more effective than the same drug in a cream base.

Pastes

There are ointments to which zinc oxide has been added, providing a stiffer consistency. They are used only in chronic dermatoses, e.g. psoriasis. They will remain on the skin surface for a considerable length of time and need only be applied once a day. They are not pleasant for the patient to use leading to difficulty with regular compliance.

When prescribing topical preparations, it is essential that patient be given the appropriate quantity to carry out the treatment correctly. In practice, it is useless to prescribe a standard 30 g tube of ointment for a patient with extensive skin disease! The prescriber must assess the area of body surface affected by the disease. As a guide, it takes approximately 30 g of cream or ointment to cover the entire body surface of an average adult. Thus, if it is estimated that 30 per cent of the skin is involved with the disease, then 10 g will be required at each application; if the preparation has to be applied twice daily, the patient will require 20 g per day or 140 g per week. Patients often ask how much ointment or cream should they apply to their rashes; it is difficult to give a clear and concise response. Drug companies are now making containers with instructions stating that a given 'length' of cream from the container will be sufficient for a given area, e.g. forearm or leg.

Topical steroids

These are the most widely used topical drugs in dermatology. Steroids have many actions, but how they work in an individual disease is not always fully understood. They have potent anti-inflammatory activity; they break down collagen and inhibit fibroblast activity; they also suppress the body's reaction to infections. They may affect factors controlling cell division and influence a large number of processes in the immune system. An important point to remember is that, if the dermatosis does not improve with topical steroids, then the possibility of an infective disorder, whether bacterial, viral or fungal, should be considered.

In recent years topical steroids have received a great deal of adverse publicity because of side effects, and patients are now often reluctant to use them. These side effects are usually avoidable and arise because physicians fail to appreciate the wide range of activity of the various topical steroid preparations available.

The steroids used in topical preparations can be assayed and their strength compared with 1 per cent hydrocortisone. From the practical point of view, it is convenient to assign the multitude of available topical steroid drugs into four groups so that one can learn about one from each group, which is all that is necessary to know. To appreciate the wide range of steroid activity available, the comparative strengths of steroids are given in Table 5.1, where the strength of hydrocortisone is equivalent to 1 unit of steroid activity.

Apart from knowing the strength of the steroid and the base required for the drug, the site to which the drug is to be applied is also important due to the variation in skin thickness and moisture. Thus, the thinner the skin, the less connective tissue present and, therefore, the greater the risk of clinical damage to the skin. The face, particularly the eyelids, and genitalia are probably the areas with the thinnest skin; as a rule, only group I steroids should be used at these sites. There is increased moisture in the intertriginous areas, which hydrates the epidermis and increases the absorption of drug into the dermis. Thus, in the intertriginous areas, only group I and II steroids should be used. These are only general guidelines as there are instances when a skin disorder on the face or genitalia has not responded to weak (i.e. group I or II) steroids. Stronger steroids will then be necessary and justified, although there should be close supervision of the patient. In general, group III and IV topical steroids should not be given on repeat prescriptions without the physician first seeing the patient.

In clinical practice, it is often necessary to give large quantities of steroid preparations in the treatment of chronic dermatoses. In these cases, it is often cheaper to dilute a group III or IV steroid with a suitable diluent. Which diluent depends on which proprietary preparation is to be prescribed. The appropriate diluent can be found in the *External Diluent Directory*. It is best to learn one diluent for one particular steroid ointment and another for one particular cream, and keep to them. Recently, the pharmaceutical industry has realised the need for large quantities of group III topical steroids and are supplying already diluted preparations.

Side effects of topical steroids

The clinical side effects are proportional to the strength of steroid used and duration of use,

Table 5.1 Comparative strengths of steroids.

Group	Strength (units)	Example (percentage)
I	1	Hydrocortisone (1)
II	25	Clobetasol butyrate (0.05)
III	100	Betamethasone 17-valerate (0.1)
IV	600	Clobetasol propionate (0.05)

and are also influenced by skin thickness and skin moisture. Steroids suppress the formation of new collagen and cause atrophy of the existing collagen, which gives rise to a variety of clinical appearances. The skin becomes thin and wrinkled, and the subcutaneous veins become prominent. Purpura may develop at sites of minor trauma, particularly on the backs of the hands and forearms and on the legs. Striae may develop, particularly in the intertriginous areas due to greater absorption of the steroid, although non-intertriginous skin may also be affected. Where the skin is particularly thin, e.g. on the face, telangiectasia may appear. Acne may be induced by the use of group III or IV topical steroids.

If topical steroids are used for fungal or bacterial infections, they may mask the usual clinical presentation and lead to diagnostic difficulties. This is particularly so with fungal infections of the skin in which the scaling and annular configuration is lost. Viral infections, particularly herpes simplex infection, may spread if topical steroids are used in the management of the condition; the obverse of this is the benefit of topical steroids in eczema herpeticum.

System side effects following the use of topical steroids are extremely rare. The side effects are proportional to the potency of the topical steroid times the quantity of steroid used. Thus, the risk is greater when potent steroids are used over large areas of skin. The most common side effect is suppression of the adrenal-pituitary axis. There are a few reports of Cushing's syndrome and even diabetes mellitus being precipitated by topical steroids.

Topical antibiotics

These are used less frequently than in the past. Many topical antibiotics (particularly neomycin and soframycin) are potential sensitizers, and the risk of strains of bacteria developing resistance to these antibiotics has also contributed to the decline in their use.

Fusidic acid and mupirocin have a low incidence of sensitization and are effective against superficial staphylococcal infections. Topical antibiotics should be avoided on chronic leg ulcers as there is an increased risk of sensitization.

Topical antihistamines and topical local anaesthetic preparations

These have no part to play in the routine treatment of skin disease. They are potential sensitizers, and topical steroids are more effective in controlling inflammation and irritation associated with epidermal disorders.

Tar preparations

These still have a definite part to play in the management of some patients with psoriasis. They may occasionally be helpful in persistent eczematous lesions. In psoriasis, crude coal tar is usually used at a concentration of 5 per cent in an ointment base (soft paraffin) or paste (Lassar's paste). Fifteen per cent coal tar solution in emulsifying ointment BP is helpful in the treatment of chronic eczematous lesions. It should be applied in liberal quantities to the trunk and limbs prior to bathing, and the use of soap should be avoided. When this preparation is used, the patient should stay in the bath for 15 minutes and use the ointment as a soap substitute as it has some cleansing properties.

Potassium permanganate soaks

At a dilution of 1:8000, potassium permanganate solution is effective in helping to control acute inflammatory dermatoses, e.g. weeping or blistering eczematous lesions, or fungal infections.

Magenta paint

This is a relatively old-fashioned remedy, but is often helpful in controlling a dermatosis affecting intertriginous areas. It has mild antifungal, antibacterial, anticandidal and astringent properties.

Topical antifungal preparations

There has been a significant increase in the number of topical antifungal preparations over the last few years. One should become familiar with a limited number and learn the spectrum of their activity and their cost.

Nystatin is only effective against yeasts and has no activity against dermatophytes (ringworm fungi).

Imidazoles are broad-spectrum agents active against yeasts (candida), dermatophytes and pityrosporum orbiculare (the fungus causing pityriasis versicolor), and corynebacterium minutissimum (erythrasma).

Terbinafine is effective against dermatophytes and pityrosporum orbiculare.

Aluminium chloride

An alcoholic solution of 25 per cent aluminium chloride hexahydrate is an effective agent in inhibiting sweating, and is very useful for essential hyperhidrosis involving the axillae and, to some extent, the palms and soles. In the axillae, the solution need only be used once or twice a week at night whereas, on the soles, daily treatment may be necessary. It is also now used as a convenient haemostasis agent.

Keratolytics

These are chemicals which disrupt keratinous protein. They are most commonly used in acne to break down excess keratin around the pilosebaceous orifice. The most commonly used keratolytics are salicylic acid and benzoyl peroxide. The strength may vary according to the type of problem treated. They are usually used in a lotion or cream base. In higher strengths, salicylic acid is used to break down wart virus structure.

PUVA (psoralen-ultraviolet A) treatment

Psoralens are naturally occurring substances found in plants but, recently, they have also been synthesized. Psoralens are potent photosensitizers and, in the presence of UV light, they also have a number of actions on cellular function. The combination of psoralens and UV light has been shown to stimulate melanocytes, impair cell division of epidermal cells, and affect the function of Langerhans cells and lymphocytes, thereby altering immune reactions.

Lamps emitting only long-wave (320–400 nm) ultraviolet light (UVA) are used for treatment with psoralens as medium-wave (90–320 nm) ultraviolet light (UVB) is responsible for the sunburn effect of UV light. Thus, by omitting UVB, the risk of sunburn is removed. However, a phototoxic reaction may occur with high doses of UVA and psoralens that is similar to a sunburn reaction. Thus, PUVA treatment is always begun with a small dose of UVA which is gradually increased only if there is no burning.

The psoralen normally used in PUVA treatment is 8-methoxypsoralen, and the dose depends on body weight. The drug has to be taken 2 hours before the patient is irradiated with UVA. Treatment is usually carried out three times a week. Focal topical PUVA may be used for local or regional diseases.

PUVA was originally used for the treatment of psoriasis, but is now also used for vitiligo, refractory eczema, lichen planus, alopecia areata and cutaneous T-cell lymphoma (mycosis fungoides). In vitiligo, the action is on the melanocytes but, in the other conditions, the clinical effects are obtained by an action on cells of the immune system and epithelial 'turnover'.

Side effects

A number of side effects of PUVA have been noticed. The most common is gastric irritation from the drug, which may be eased by taking the psoralen with food, particularly milk. Metoclopromide is also helpful and should be taken with the psoralens. If the nausea persists, a change from the commonly used 8-methoxypsoralen to 5 methoxypsoralen may stop or decrease the nausea.

If the dose of UVA light is too high, there may be redness and soreness of the skin and, in severe cases, blistering of the skin.

A rare side effect seen mainly in middle-aged men is itching and hyperesthesia over the upper trunk. If PUVA is given for any length of time, the effects as seen with overexposure to sunlight may occur, e.g. lentigos and degeneration of elastic tissue.

A UV light is potentially carcinogenic, there is a risk of skin cancers with PUVA. However, so far, the only increase of skin cancers reported is that of squamous cell carcinomata on the male genitalia. Therefore, male patients are now advised to cover the genitalia with appropriate clothing during treatment.

Oral retinoids

These drugs have been introduced into dermatology over the last decade. They are derivatives of vitamin A (retinol). It has long been known that vitamin A is necessary for the growth, differentiation and maintenance of epithelial tissues. Vitamin A has been used in a number of dermatological conditions over the years, but was not particularly effective and, in high doses, is toxic, causing the hypervitaminosis A syndrome, including raised cerebrospinal fluid pressure, hepatomegaly, splenomegaly, dry scaly skin, dryness of the mucous membranes, bone pain and anorexia.

Retinoids have long been synthesized and have been shown to have biological effects on many epithelia, including the skin. There are two retinoids in current use — isotretinoin and acitretin. The latter drug is mainly used in psoriasis, Darier's disease and some of the ichthyoses. Isotretinoin is used mainly for acne. Retinoids have been of considerable benefit to dermatological practice, and newer retinoids with other actions are likely to be developed. Unfortunately, as with all drugs, retinoids are not without side effects. The most common side effects are cheilitis (dry cracked lips), dry skin, dry mucosal surfaces, hair loss and mild eczematous patches. The most serious side effect of retinoids is teratogenicity. Because of this, women of childbearing age must be warned; adequate contraception is essential. Patients should also be told that, although it takes 1 month for isotretinoin to be excreted from the body after cessation of treatment, it takes 2 years for excretion of acitretin.

If retinoids are given for psoriasis or genodermatoses, they may be taken for long periods or even indefinitely, and there are a number of possible long-term side effects. Retinoids tend to raise serum lipids and, thus, fasting lipids should be checked before commencing long-term treatment and then at 6-month intervals. There is also a slight risk of hepatotoxicity and, therefore, liver function must be monitored. Retinoids may also affect the musculoskeletal system. Transient arthralgia and muscle pain may occur particularly after strenuous exercise. Premature closing of the epiphysis has been reported in children. Finally, although rare, the diffuse idiopathic interstitial skeletal hyperostosis (DISH) syndrome may occur, with ossification of ligaments and accretion of bone onto vertebral bodies, raising the question of periodic radiographic examinations, the place of which is still to be determined. How retinoids work and why they should be effective in diseases with different pathologies is not known but, with more research and a better understanding of the disease processes, retinoids are likely to be important drugs in the future.

Cyclosporin

In dermatology, cyclosporin was first used for psoriasis and, more recently, for atopic eczema. It has a specific action on activated CD4 T-lymphocytes. Thus, skin diseases which are mediated by these cells should respond to cyclosporin. Cyclosporin tends to be reserved for widespread and persistent disease which does not respond to other treatments. It is a highly effective drug for both psoriasis and atopic eczema. However, like most of the currently available effective treatments, there are side effects. The two most serious are nephrotoxicity and hypertension. Therefore, prior

to commencing treatment, it is essential to establish that patients have normal renal function. During treatment, both renal function and blood pressure must be monitored.

Methotrexate

This drug has been used for many years for severe psoriasis, for which it is highly effective. Immediate side effects are nausea, lethargy, gastrointestinal ulceration and bone marrow depression. The most important long-term side effect is hepatotoxicity and, thus, liver function must be monitored. Periodic liver biopsy may be necessary in long-term treatment. This is of particular benefit in acral digital pustular psoriasis.

Antifungal drugs

Griseofulvin is only effective against dermatophyte infections. It has to be taken for 1 month for skin infections, 6 weeks for scalp infections and 6–9 months for fingernail infections. It is not as effective for toenail infections. *Terbinafine* is effective against dermatophyte infections. Its main indication is toenail infections, for which it is especially effective. *Itraconazole* and *fluconazole* are broad-spectrum antibiotics effective against yeast as well as dermatophyte infections. They are also effective for nail infections when taken weekly for several months. Itraconazole has an 80 per cent chance of clearing pityriasis versicolor after 1 week of treatment.

Antihistamines

These drugs have an antipruritic action. Many of them make patients drowsy, which is useful at night but not during the day. Their main indications are in the control of pruritus and in the treatment of urticaria.

Dapsone

This sulfone has been used in the treatment of leprosy for many years. It is effective in clearing the lesions of dermatitis herpetiformis as well as in a number of other conditions with an immunological basis, particularly cutaneous vasculitis.

The main side effects are haemolysis and methaemoglobinaemia.

Sunscreens

Ultraviolet light is that part of the solar spectrum which tends to cause most skin problems. Ultraviolet light is divided into UVC (short waves that are screened by the ozone layer), UVB (medium waves) and UVA (long waves).

UVB is responsible for the sunburn effect, but UVA may cause a number of photodermatoses. UVB is definitely carcinogenic and UVA is probably likewise. UVA is thought to play an important part in photo-ageing as it damages the elastic tissue of the dermis and causes wrinkles.

Most sunscreens currently in use are absorbent, i.e. they work by absorbing the energy of ultraviolet light. They are effective against UVB, but have little or no action against UVA. The main compounds used in absorbent sunscreens are esters of para-aminobenzoic acid, esters of cinnamic acid and benzophenones.

Substances which reflect UV light are protective against UVB and UVA. Examples are titanium dioxide and zinc oxide.

The skin protection factor (SPF) of sunscreens refers to its ability to block out UVB light. The SPF number is the ratio of the time needed to produce minimal erythema with the sunscreen (Tp) compared with no protection (T); thus, SPF = Tp/T. None of the sunscreens are totally effective in screening out either UVB or UVA.

PHYSICAL AND SURGICAL TREATMENTS

During the last 20 years there has been a great revolution in the practice of skin surgery by specialists who previously would have done no surgery; or no more than the simplest biopsies and non-excisional physical procedures. At the time of writing, in the Western world all trainee dermatologists now undertake mandatory skin surgery training to a very detailed level; also dermatology surgery nurse practitioners are extending their skills into excisional operations whilst podiatrists are expanding the range of skin surgical procedures that they can be licensed to undertake. The purpose of this section is to give a general outline of procedures capable of being used at the overlap of the dermatological surgeon, plastic surgeon, surgical nurse practitioner and podiatrist.

Local anaesthetics

Principles and types

The prime considerations are effectiveness, rapid action and relative freedom from toxicity and sensitization. These qualities are found in lignocaine hydrochloride (lidocaine), an amide-type local anaesthetic, which is the agent of choice for most dermatologists. Procaine (ester of *p*-aminobenzoic acid) is recommended chiefly by anaesthetists because of its lower toxicity, but the amounts used by dermatologists in standard procedures are usually small, and its cross-reactivity with other drugs of the *p*-aminobenzoic acid ester type is a strong disincentive to its use. Of three other preparations of the same general amino group as lignocaine, mepivacaine and bupivacaine are similar but have a more sustained action (up to 480 minutes with adrenaline), whereas prilocaine has a rather briefer effect (60–400 minutes).

Methods

Local anaesthesia may be achieved topically using either amethocaine cream (Ametop) or a eutectic lignocaine-prilocaine cream (EMLA), or by local infiltration. Both EMLA and Ametop are applied under occlusion, the former for at least 2 hours and the latter for 1 hour. Other methods or anaesthesia include field block (Figure 5.1) or regional anaesthesia which produce temporary interruption of sensory nerve conductivity in a given area. Field block involves infiltration of local anaesthetic at several points around the lesion to be excised, and nerve block involves infiltration close to the nerve supplying the operative field. The choice of which type of local anaesthetic to use depends not only on the method of anaesthesia and the site and expected duration of operation but also on the patient's general condition and the physician's own preference and experience.

To achieve 'regional' anaesthesia of digits the technique known as 'ring block' is used — all four digital nerves are injected by this method (Figure 5.2). To avoid vasospasm of all the adjacent digital arteries (and possible gangrene) local anaesthetic without adrenaline must be used for ring block.

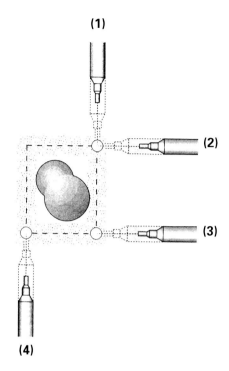

Figure 5.1

Field block anaesthesia prior to excision. **(1)** The first injection is given subcutaneously (use a long needle to avoid having repeated punctures; warn patients that they will feel a prick and then a burning sensation). **(2)** Once the insertion site is numb, advance the needle along one edge of the area to be anaesthetized, slowly injecting the anaesthetic (choose the side closest to the origin of the sensory nerve innervating the area). **(3)** Once the next corner is numb, insert the needle again. **(4)** Repeat until a ring of skin around the area is anaesthetized.

The maximum recommended dosage for lignocaine with adrenaline (epinephrine) is 7 mg/kg or approximately 50 ml of a 1 per cent lignocaine solution. In practice, most skin surgeons use substantially less. Children should receive smaller amounts of more dilute preparations. Before injecting any local anaesthetic,

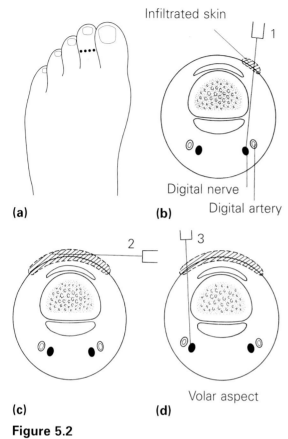

Figure 5.2

(a) Site of ring block, **(b–d)** successive positions of needle.

it is a wise precaution to aspirate first. This should be mandatory when attempting nerve blocks.

Other anaesthetic agents include the following:

- Ethylchloride, dichlorotetrafluorethane (Freon), solid carbon dioxide snow and liquid nitrogen spray give short-lived periods of anaesthesia with refrigeration. These are suitable for the incision of small cysts, abscesses or superficial skin lesions, and for the curettage of multiple small warts or milia.
- The anaesthetic effect of antihistamines can be used when hypersensitivity to other

agents is present. Diphenhydramine hydrochloride as a 1 per cent solution is suitable.
- The injection into the skin of sufficient normal saline to cause a weal may be used to produce an anaesthetic effect.
- Benzodiazepines such as intravenous diazepam (2.5–10 mg) are useful to allay anxiety, particularly in children, but are not specifically anaesthetic at 'sedative' doses. However, small procedures such as the removal of a molluscum contagiosum can often be carried out with less distress following its administration. Topical local anaesthesia may be adequate for minor lesions in children.

Cryosurgery

The earliest freezing agent used in the 'modern' treatment of skin diseases was the salt-ice mixture (-20°C) advocated by Arnott in 1851. By 1913, the clinical effectiveness of liquid air and solid carbon dioxide (carbon dioxide snow) was well known. Increasing knowledge in the field of cryobiology, together with the development of sophisticated cryoprobes and liquid gas jets, has led to a great increase in the use of cryosurgery during the last 30 years.

Liquid nitrogen is now most commonly used throughout the world; its boiling point is -196°C. Nitrous oxide gas is also used as a refrigerant in closed probe systems (applying the Joule–Thompson effect), giving a working temperature of -70°C.

Clinical methods

Carbon dioxide snow is little used now, but if no other refrigerant is available satisfactory results can be obtained, mainly for benign lesions. It is made by releasing gas from a cylinder into a chamois leather bag, and the solid 'snow' is then transferred to a plastic funnel tube in which it is compressed. Alternatively, small cylinders of gas may be discharged through a narrow opening into a collecting tube. Such apparatus is useful for superficial lesions; deeper destruction can only be achieved by applying greater pressure with special applicators.

Liquid nitrogen is universally available owing to its widespread use in industry, hospital and research establishments. It is very cheap. The liquid is unstable at room temperature, but 1 litre stored in an unsealed (Dewar) flask will last a full day and treat 50–60 patients. Cotton-wool swabs or copper discs are dipped into the liquid and applied to the skin for 5–30 seconds. Liquid nitrogen sprays and probes are now commercially available for use when greater tissue destruction is required, and have become standard equipment in clinical practice; this type of 'accurate', more destructive equipment is mandatory if preneoplastic and malignant lesions are to be treated (Figure 5.3).

Nitrous oxide cryoprobes are also available. The gas is easily obtained because of its use in anaesthesia. This refrigerant is less appropriate than liquid nitrogen for treating malignancy.

Clinical uses

A wide spectrum of skin lesions has been treated with freezing. Table 5.2 shows a list of many of the conditions that may occur on the feet in which cure has been reported. The simplicity and speed of cryosurgery treatment make it particularly attractive for dermatological practice. It must be stressed that, for most lesions in Table 5.2 other modes of treatment may be equally effective; one always has to balance the advantages and disadvantages of each treatment method for each lesion in each patient.

Lesions that are superficial, benign or flat can be treated by the liquid nitrogen cotton-wool swab method if the standard spray or probe equipment is not available. To obtain cure of preneoplastic and neoplastic conditions, the lower temperature and most consistently destructive properties of liquid nitrogen spray or probe are desirable.

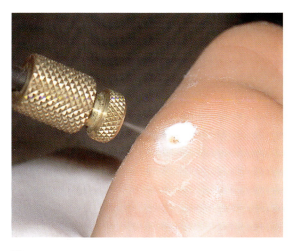

Figure 5.3
Cryosurgery (liquid nitrogen spray) in action.

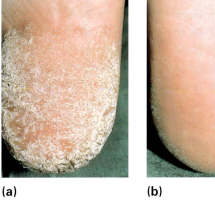

(a)   **(b)**
Figure 5.4
(a) Large mosaic (viral) wart.
(b) Four months later, following six applications of liquid nitrogen spray.

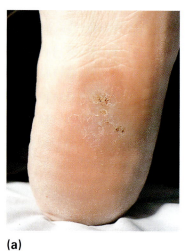 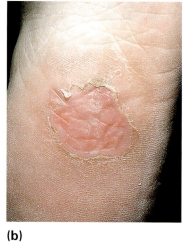 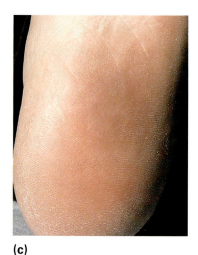

(a)   **(b)**   **(c)**

Figure 5.5

(a) Grouped warts.
(b) Four weeks after treatment.
(c) Sixteen weeks after treatment (courtesy of Dr EC Benton, Edinburgh, UK).

Table 5.2 Skin conditions responsive to cryosurgery.

Naevi	Pigmented
	Epidermal
Lentigo	Benign and malignant
Vascular lesions	Telangiectasia
	Spider naevus
	Pyogenic granuloma
	Pseudopyogenic granuloma
	Kaposi's sarcoma
	Haemangioma
	Lymphangioma
Keratotic and preneoplastic	Viral warts (Figures 5.4 and 5.5)
	Molluscum contagiosum
	Seborrhoeic keratosis
	Solar keratosis
	Cutaneous horn
	Keratoacanthoma
	Bowen's disease
Carcinoma	Basal cell epithelioma
	Squamous cell eipthelioma
Cysts	Epidermal
	Synovial
	Myxoid cyst
Toe	Ingrowing nail (Figure 5.6)

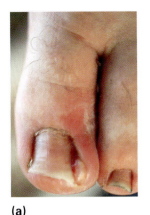
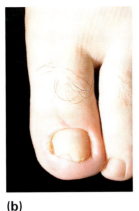

(a)   **(b)**

Figure 5.6

(a) Ingrowing toenail with epithelialized periungual granulation tissue.
(b) Eight weeks after a single freeze-thaw cycle (20 seconds freeze after ice formation) to the abnormal area.

Side effects

Pain is minimal compared with surgery and is usually transient, due to the anaesthetizing effect of freezing. Oedema is not uncommon in 'lax' tissue. Haemorrhagic blisters may occur. It is important to note that blister formation is not necessary for the cure of lesions such as viral warts.

Sun-damaged and senile atrophic skin, and areas previously treated with topical steroids or X-irradiation, are more likely to blister or become necrotic after freezing. Skin necrosis is a desirable part of the treatment of neoplastic and many preneoplastic lesions, and several weeks may elapse before healing is complete after 'tumour' treatment schedules. Hypopigmentation is common after low-temperatures liquid nitrogen cryosurgery (probe or jet), particularly in dark-skinned patients. Temporary postinflammatory hyperpigmentation is to be expected following less severe freezing. Paraesthesiae and, rarely, anaesthesia occur, and may be trouble-

some because of the local effect of freezing on nerve endings. Care must be taken to avoid damage to major nerves, as distal anaesthesia and motor paralysis may occur; however, these rare effects are temporary. Adventitious glands are sensitive to freezing.

Curettage

Benign lesions

Curettage of viral warts, like all therapies, is not totally effective (Figures 5.7, 5.8). The treatment is painful and there is a risk of scarring and recurrence. Solitary warts on the face of adults can usually be removed effectively using curettage. Otherwise, curettage of viral warts should only be performed when other methods have failed. Plantar warts may be removed by curettage but the local anaesthetic injections

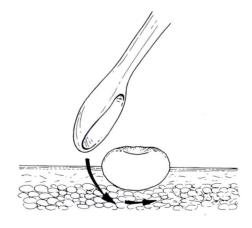

Figure 5.7

Curettage: soft, abnormal tissue is easily distinguished from the firm normal dermis. Fibrosing or scarred tumours cannot be removed with a curette.

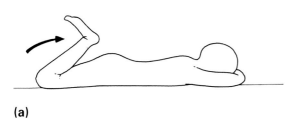

(a)

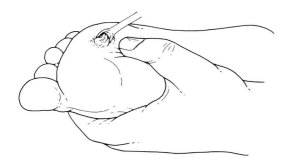

(b)

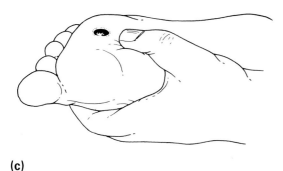

(c)

Figure 5.8

Curettage of a plantar wart.
(a) The patient is prone with the foot elevated.
(b) The wart is anaesthetized and removed by curettage while the operator's thumb applies firm pressure to prevent blood obscuring the field.
(c) A topical haemostatic agent is applied before digital pressure is released.

are painful unless nerve-block anaesthesia is successful. Recurrences can be a problem, as patients are unlikely to tolerate repeat treatment. Curettage is probably justifiable in painful, solitary, plantar warts, which have not responded to other therapies, although the patient should be warned of the slight risk of permanent, potentially painful, scar formation. Periungual warts are difficult to curette off and curettage should only be employed as a last resort; the nail may have to be avulsed to allow adequate access for curettage. Multiple digital warts should not be treated by curettage unless all else has failed. Multiple seborrhoeic warts are best treated by cryosurgery. Solitary warts or those that have not responded to cryosurgery can be curetted off if necessary.

Other lesions such a pyogenic granulomas and actinic keratoses are commonly treated using curettage. Curettage is only possible if the material being scraped off is more frail than the surrounding skin, or where there is a natural cleavage plane between the lesion and the surrounding normal tissue. The resulting shallow wound heals by a combination of wound shrinkage and re-epithelialization from the follicular and edge epithelium. Tense and fix the numbed skin using the finger and thumb. Scrape off the lesion with the edge of a sharp spoon or ring curettage until a smooth surface remains. On mobile areas, first fulgurize or incize the wart margin to obtain a plane of cleavage. Stop bleeding using either cautery, electrodesiccation or a chemical haemostatic agent. Do not use alcohol-based skin-cleansing solutions when using cautery or electrodesiccation because of the risk of fire.

Intraepidermal carcinoma (Bowen's disease)

Intraepidermal carcinoma, especially on the lower leg, can be treated by curettage.

Although all wounds at this site heal slowly, particularly if there is co-existing oedema or poor peripheral circulation, curettage is possibly superior to radiotherapy, 5-fluorouracil or cryosurgery, as the extent of treatment is more predictably determined by the operator.

Electrosurgery

Electrosurgery includes electrodesiccation, electrofulguration, cutting diathermy and electrolysis. Coagulation or tissue destruction is produced by the heat created as the electrical current passes through the tissue. Although not strictly an electrosurgical technique, electrocautery is usually also included because of its development from the age-old method of using heat in the form of hot oils, cautery irons, etc., to control bleeding.

Electrocautery (syn: cautery; hot-wire cautery)

The cautery machine power output should be controllable so that the tip temperature can be adjusted rather than being dependent on the battery power. A variety of tips are available. The beaded tip is best for haemostasis after curettage and shave biopsy; this should be just hot enough to char a cotton swab, but not red hot as the platinum tip may melt. If the beaded tip drags on the tissue as it is drawn across the wound, the tip temperature is too low. After use, any remaining debris should be burnt off by briefly allowing the tip to become red hot. The needle-like end of the cold point cautery tip is heated, by conduction, via a wire coil, and is used to treat spider naevi. The flat blade can be used for pedunculated lesions or shave excision, but has to be glowing red hot to cut

through tissue, producing a heating artefact on the excised material. Furthermore, the red-hot blade has to be quickly passed through the skin to avoid excessive heat damage at the wound site, so the direction and depth of the cut cannot be adjusted easily and the blade may accidentally cut or burn deeper into the tissue than required.

Electrosurgical diathermy (syn: cold cautery; hyfrecation)

Electrosurgical equipment converts domestic alternating current into high-frequency alternating current. When this passes through a high-resistance medium, such as the skin and fat, heat is produced resulting in tissue coagulation, desiccation or cutting, depending on the electrical waveform. A highly damped waveform (i.e. intermittent pulses), results in electrodesiccation/fulguration, a continuous waveform produces a cutting effect and coagulation is produced by a slightly damped waveform. There is overlap between these effects.

Unipolar/monoterminal bipolar diathermy

Apart from the waveform produced, electrosurgery equipment also varies in the way it discharges and collects the current. Unipolar (monopolar) current is delivered via an active electrode, usually a needle or ball tip, resulting in a high concentration of current at the electrode tip. The current disperses through the patient's body and is collected via a dispersive (syn: indifferent, passive, return, ground) electrode with a large surface area. The current density falls with increasing distance from the active electrode and there is minimal risk of tissue damage as the current is collected over the large area of the dispersive electrode. If, due to faulty application or equipment, there is only a small area of skin/electrode contact, a burn may occur at the dispersive electrode. Also, if the current is channelled at narrow points along its path, for example the penis, an area of high-current density leading to tissue damage can occur. Bipolar electrodes avoid these hazards by producing and collecting the current via a pair of forceps so that current only travels in the tissue held between the tips of the forceps, not through the whole patient. Monoterminal electrosurgical equipment (e.g. Birtcher Hyfrecator) produces a high-voltage, low-amperage current, and is designed to be used without a dispersive electrode. This is probably the commonest machine used in skin surgery practice. There is, however, a risk of a small but painful discharge occurring between the patient and the operator or some other grounded or earthed point, for example the edge of a metal table, if the patient is lying on an electrically insulated couch. This can be prevented by maintaining a large area of skin contact between the operator and patient during use, or using a dispersive electrode.

Electrodesiccation/ electrofulguration

This is produced using a monoterminal or unipolar electrode. Electrodesiccation ('electrical drying') occurs when the needle remains in contact with the skin and no spark occurs. Because the current concentration is greater at the point of contact, the tissue damage is slightly deeper compared with electrofulguration ('like lightning'). During the latter, the needle tip is not in contact with the skin and a spark jumps between the skin and the needle, but its energy is spread over a greater area. The resulting heat causes superficial damage

to the tissues and is an effective way of stopping bleeding from capillaries. Various needle tips have been developed for specific circumstances. Because of the risk of virus transmission, a different clean needle must be used for each patient.

Using an electrosurgical unit may temporarily stop a pacemaker working, so that the patient's heart may stop beating briefly if there is no underlying cardiac rhythm. Alternatively, the pacemaker may deviate from a demand to a fixed-rate mode as this is not affected by the electrosurgical current. The effect lasts only as long as the unit is being operated. When diathermy finishes, the pacemaker reverts to normal function. There are also anecdotal reports of the pacemaker failing shortly after electrosurgery. Diathermy used directly over a pacemaker may rarely cause its permanent reprogramming, but permanent inhibition is very rare. All pacemakers, particularly older versions, are vulnerable. All types of electrosurgical equipment, apart from electrocautery, can cause the problem. Bipolar diathermy is least hazardous, and where possible should be used in preference to monoterminal or monopolar diathermy. With both monopolar and bipolar diathermy, only short bursts (less than 5 seconds) should be used, the patient's heart rate should be monitored and resuscitation equipment should be available. Diathermy should not be performed within 15 cm of the heart, the pacemaker or its leads. If monopolar diathermy has to be used, the path from the active electrode (diathermy tip) to the dispersive electrode must also be at least 15 cm from the heart, the pacemaker and its leads. Electrosurgery is widely used in different modes and for different lesions:

- as part of the process of curettage and electrosurgery for superficial skin lesions and tumours
- focal vascular lesions
- benign papillomas
- Small seborrhoeic and viral warts.

Excisional surgical procedures including biopsies

Whilst the more subtle and complex skin and nail procedures are always likely to require the detail, training and experience of medical graduates, there are many operations that nurse practitioners and podiatrists have already been trained to undertake. What follows will be limited to the 'interface' between the specialists stated above.

Skin biopsy techniques

A good skin biopsy can provide valuable information, but a biopsy that is too small or too superficial, or one that is taken from a lesion that is too old or too young, may be useless.

Shave biopsy

Indications

- Benign superficial epidermal lesions, e.g. seborrhoeic keratoses, actinic keratoses
- Benign intradermal naevi may be partially removed, but hyperpigmentation may recur and hairs nearly always regrow.

The disadvantage is that deep dermis and fat are not sampled. After skin antiseptic cleaning and local anaesthetic injection a thin section is removed using a large scalpel blade (no. 22) held parallel to the skin. The surface should remain slightly raised. If nodules are shaved down to skin level, they heal with a depressed scar, which may be more unsightly than the original lesion. Haemostasis is obtained using pressure and a topical haemostatic agent.

Punch biopsy

The punch is a cylindrical cutting instrument which is available in varying diameters. A 4 mm punch provides an adequate tissue sample for histological examination. In reality, this 'circular knife' is twisted into the skin rather than directly punched into the tissue.

The main indications for punch biopsy

- To obtain a tissue sample from possible tumours before definitive treatment
- To remove small lesions
- To provide small amounts of tissue for direct immunofluorescence or electron microscopy, or culture.

This method of biopsy is rapid but there are some limitations:

- The sample is small and may not be representative of the whole lesions. An elliptical biopsy through a tumour demonstrates the architecture more clearly
- A punch biopsy does not show the transition from normal to abnormal skin
- Fat frequently sheers off. A punch biopsy is therefore unsuitable for sampling lesions primarily in subcutaneous tissue
- It may be difficult to orientate a small punch biopsy after fixation, so some pathologists prefer an elliptical specimen.

The technique

- The skin is cleaned and anaesthetized
- The skin is held stretched at 90° to the natural wrinkle lines while the punch is

inserted, pushed downward and twisted back and forth. A slight 'give' is felt as the punch goes through the dermis. It is important to push the punch deep enough to obtain some underlying fat and provide an adequate tissue sample

- The punch is withdrawn. The core of tissue may come out with the punch. If it does not, the base can be cut with a pair of scissors or scalpel blade, while the surrounding skin is depressed to prevent blood obscuring the field. It may be necessary to lift up the specimen to separate it deeply
- The specimen should be gently removed with forceps or the scissors
- The circular defect will relax into an ellipse. Firm pressure will soon stop any bleeding. The defect can be closed with an absorbable suture and/or steristrips.

Elliptical biopsy

The biopsy may be incisional or excisional (see page 151). The main indications are:

- To examine the transition from normal to abnormal skin
- To examine the overall architecture of a lesion, e.g. keratoacanthoma: a biopsy should always be taken right across the tumour, bisecting it
- To obtain samples from subcutaneous tissue, e.g. erythema nodosum, nodular vasculitis
- To obtain additional tissue for culture, direct immunofluorescence or electron microscopy. A single elliptical biopsy may be preferable to several small punch biopsies.

The technique of incisional biopsy

- The biopsy should extend from normal skin into the centre of the lesion, run parallel to the wrinkle lines and measure at least 1 cm in length
- The incision lines are marked with gentian violet of Bonney's blue
- The skin is cleaned and anaesthetized
- The skin is incised vertically down to subcutaneous tissues using a no. 15 scalpel blade. A second incision is made almost parallel to the first, meeting it at the corners, forming a narrow ellipse. The incisions must be vertical. If the wound edge is sloped there is less subcutaneous tissue removed, the specimen is unsatisfactory and the wound is more difficult to close
- The specimen is lifted up gently by one corner. The base is cut with a scalpel as it is peeled back
- The wound is closed with interrupted sutures.

Elliptical excision technique

Principles of excisional biopsy are essentially the same as elliptical excision (page 156).

Important practical points include:

- Remember to photograph any unusual lesion before removing it
- Plan the investigations, obtain fixatives and culture mediums and if necessary talk to the pathologist so that you know how much tissue you need
- Choose the lesion:
  (a) In most disorders, biopsy a fully developed lesion that is not damaged by scratching, minor trauma or secondarily infection
  (b) The edge is often the most active part of the lesion, e.g. annular erythemas

(c) Bullous disorders: biopsy a fresh bulla less than 24 hours old, or a pre-bullous 'urticarial' lesion.

Local anaesthetic

Inject it just under the skin to prevent the fluid in the skin distorting the anatomy. Lignocaine and adrenaline will cause mast cells to degranulate. In suspected urticaria pigmentosa, plain lignocaine should be injected around the biopsy site, not directly into it.

Nail biopsy

Indications

This is indicated for the diagnosis of nail dystrophies and tumours. Diabetes, scleroderma and peripheral vascular disease are relative contra-indications to nail surgery.

Technique

A complete digital ('ring') block is performed at the base of the digit, using 2 per cent lignocaine without adrenaline (see Figure 5.2). A tourniquet prevents bleeding. This should be removed within 20 minutes.

There are several methods of taking a nail biopsy (see Figure 5.9).

Punch biopsy

Indication

Local tumour of the bed or matrix. This technique provides a small sample of the nail plate and the underlying bed or matrix, with very good cosmetic results (Figure 5.9a, b). The latter is clearly very important for non-malignant diseases and lesions.

A 3 mm punch is passed through the nail plate into the nail bed or matrix. A thick nail plate may need prior soaking in water to soften it. The nail over the nail matrix is softer than that over the nail bed. A scalpel is used to cut to the base of the biopsy and the specimen is removed. The depth of the biopsy is to bone level since the nail apparatus have no subcutaneous fat layer.

Elliptical biopsy of the nail bed

Indication

The technique for excision or biopsy of tumours (Figure 5.9c) involves:

- the nail plate is separated from the nail bed and cut away to expose the lesion
- a narrow longitudinal ellipse of tissue is excised
- the edges are closed with dexon.

Longitudinal nail biopsy

Indication

Nail dystrophies. The specimen provides simultaneous information about the whole length of the nail apparatus including the nail matrix, bed and plate. Samples can be sent for culture.

Two parallel incisions are made laterally in the nail plate, extending from the proximal nail fold to the tip of the finger (Figure 5.9d). The width between these incisions should not exceed 3 mm or the nail may remain split. The

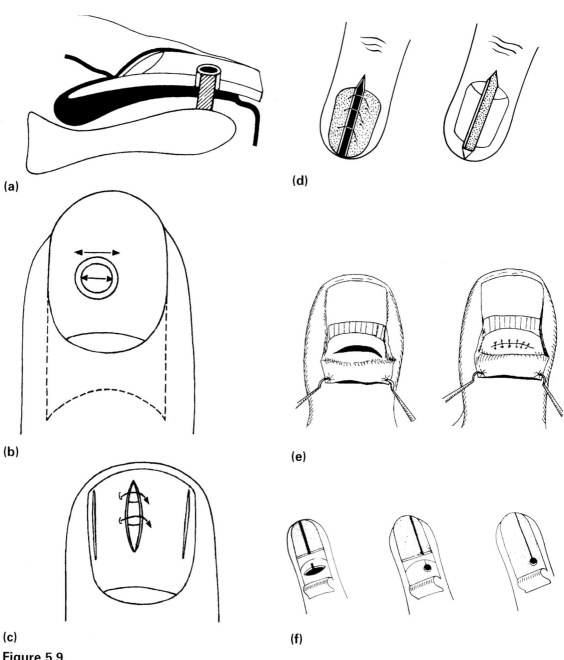

(a)

(b)

(c)

(d)

(e)

(f)

Figure 5.9

Nail biopsy techniques.
(a, b) Punch biopsy.
(c)   Elliptical biopsy of nail bed.
(d)   Longitudinal nail apparatus biopsy.
(e, f) Elliptical and punch matrix biopsy.

incisions should be carried down to, but not into, bone.

Two short horizontal incisions join the longitudinal incisions and complete the rectangle. The rectangular specimen is gently dissected off the bone using sharp, curved, iris scissors. The wound is closed with widely spaced 4/0 nylon sutures. A pressure dressing is applied and left in place for 4–5 days. Tissue can be sent for fungal culture and histology.

Elliptical and punch matrix biopsies

These are used to investigate pigmented lesions and some nail dystrophies (Figure 5.9e, f).

Excision and direct closure

The maximum size of any lesion which can be excized and sutured directly is dependent on the mobility of the local skin. The advantages of excision include:

- the whole specimen can be submitted for histological diagnosis and completeness of excision
- patients do not require lengthy follow-up after excision as the recurrence rate following complete excision is very low
- one treatment only is necessary
- primary wound healing is usually achieved, giving a good cosmetic result.

The margins of excision should be marked prior to infiltration with local anaesthetic as this distorts the tissues.

The shape of the lesion may suggest the direction of the ellipse but, if possible, the longitudinal axis of the ellipse should lie in or parallel to a natural crease in the skin (Figures

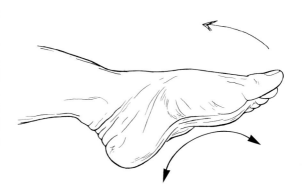

Figure 5.10

Foot must be flexed and extended at the joints to judge the lines of excision.

5.10, 5.11). The lines of excision on the foot and toes can in general be judged by flexing and extending the foot at the ankle mid-foot and toes. Natural visible skin creases may also be guides as most typically seen on the face (Figure 5.10).

Crushing tissue leads to devitalization of tissue which inevitably leads to poor healing and thus poor scars. Skin edges should be handled with care. They should never be crushed by holding with any forceps, toothed or non-toothed. Fine-toothed forceps should be used to grip the dermis or to stabilize the skin edge with pressure. A skin hook could be used instead.

A no.15 blade is useful for almost any simple excision. Lax skin should be held under tension as the cut is made. All incisions should be made vertical to the skin except in hair-bearing areas.

Undermining (3–4mm) should be carried out in all cases of excision in order to allow eversion of the wound edges when suturing. More undermining may be needed to take the tension off the wound edges. Undermining will always produce more bleeding and increase the risk of haematoma.

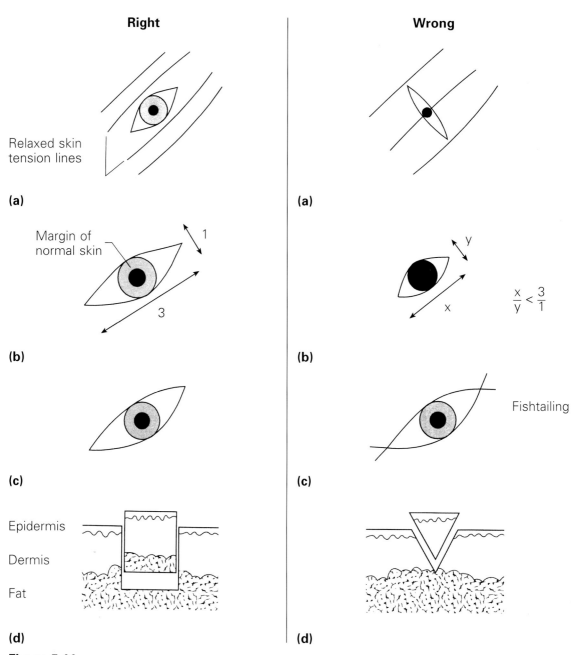

Figure 5.11

Principles of elliptical excision.
(a) Follows skin lines.
(b) Should be approximately three times as long as it is wide.
(c) Hold the blade vertically at the ends of the ellipse to prevent the incision lines crossing over.
(d) Hold the blade at 90° to the skin when cutting, to provide vertical sides.

Most bleeding can be stopped by applying pressure and waiting for a few minutes. Various methods are available to speed up the haemostatic process:

- pressure
- elevation of the limb
- clipping vessels with mosquito forceps
- tying vessels with 3/0 or 4/0 plain catgut
- bipolar diathermy.

Suturing technique

The aim of suturing is to produce accurately apposed, everted wound edges in an atraumatic manner. This should produce healing by primary intention leading to a scar of good quality. The operator should be comfortably seated with a good light source. If an assistant is available, the wound can be stretched lengthwise between two skin hooks. This helps to stabilize the skin and makes suturing easier. There are several methods of suturing wounds, but for the purposes of this book only the simple interrupted method which is most commonly used on the foot is described (Figure 5.12).

- The needle should be placed in the needle holder one-third to a half of the way along the curve from the suture material
- In the opposite hand, a pair of forceps (e.g. toothed Adson's) should be used to grip the dermis or stabilize the skin edge by applying pressure
- The needle tip should be inserted at 90° to the skin and it should be angled so as to take a larger 'bite' of the deeper part of the skin
- An equal 'bite' of skin must be taken from the outer edge of the wound and by lifting the skin edge with a hook or rolling the

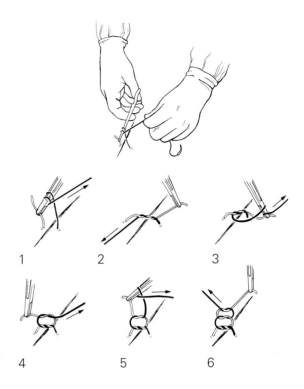

Figure 5.12

The square knot — one example of a knot used to tie a suture.

dermis outwards with a pair of toothed forceps, the deeper part of the bite will be wider and thus the skin edges will be everted (NB: Inverted wound edges will produce depressed, ugly scars.)

- Tying knots using instruments allows more control over suture tension (Figure 5.12). If the stitching is too tight, the wound edges will be strangulated and devitalized, leading to poor healing. If the stitching is too loose, the wound will gape. For a few days after the operation there will be some oedema in the wound edges and therefore stitches will apparently become tighter.

Index

Page numbers in *italic* refer to figures or tables